Unveiling Ulcerative Colitis - A Comprehensive Approach to Understanding and Management

Edited by Daniela Cornelia Lazar

Published in London, United Kingdom

Unveiling Ulcerative Colitis - A Comprehensive Approach to Understanding and Management
http://dx.doi.org/10.5772/intechopen.1001701
Edited by Daniela Cornelia Lazar

Contributors
Alen Biščanin, Bethany Malone, Bhavani Gadiraju, César Enrique Garnica Camacho, Dominik Kralj, Doris Ogresta, Griffin Bryant, Gulustan H. Babayeva, Jhansi Magisetty, Jonathan Hughes, Konul M. Kerimova, Makhir T. Ramazanov, Namig O. Isgandarov, Petra Ćaćić, Sarai Krewson, Uğur Korkmaz, Vedran Tomašić, Vijay Kondreddy, Ömer Şentürk

First published in London, United Kingdom, 2025 by IntechOpen
IntechOpen is the global imprint of INTECHOPEN LIMITED, registered in England and Wales, registration number: 11086078, 167-169 Great Portland Street, London, W1W 5PF, United Kingdom

For EU product safety concerns: IN TECH d.o.o., Prolaz Marije Krucifikse Kozulić 3, 51000 Rijeka, Croatia, info@intechopen.com or visit our website at intechopen.com.

British Library Cataloguing-in-Publication Data
A catalogue record for this book is available from the British Library

Unveiling Ulcerative Colitis - A Comprehensive Approach to Understanding and Management
Edited by Daniela Cornelia Lazar
p. cm.
Print ISBN 978-0-85466-666-9
Online ISBN 978-0-85466-665-2
eBook (PDF) ISBN 978-0-85466-745-1

If disposing of this product, please recycle the paper responsibly.

Meet the editor

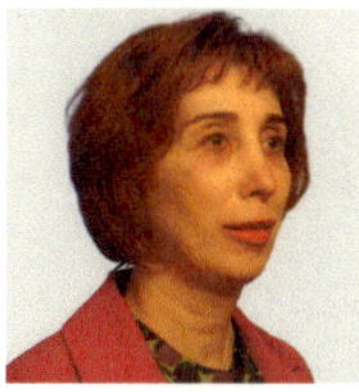

Assoc. Prof. Dr. Daniela Lazar began her career at a center of excellence in the Department of Gastroenterology and Hepatology at the University of Medicine and Pharmacy "Victor Babes" in Timişoara, Romania, where she acquired clinical skills in gastroenterology, learned the techniques of endoscopy and abdominal ultrasonography, and initiated her research activity. Besides gastroenterology, she showed interest in the oncological field and the research of gastrointestinal neoplastic conditions, especially gastric cancer. Dr. Lazar specializes in gastroenterology, medical oncology, and internal medicine. Besides her academic and teaching activities, she is involved in integrated clinical practice in the Department of Internal Medicine at the Emergency Military Clinical Hospital Timisoara. Dr. Lazar completed a Ph.D. thesis in the field of gastric cancer. She has participated in numerous national and international congresses, presenting research studies in the fields of gastroenterology, internal medicine, and digestive oncology. She has published research studies in numerous renowned international journals on angiogenesis, premalignant lesions, and prognostic factors in gastric cancer. She also published review articles regarding targeted treatments and immunotherapy in gastric cancer, as well as the impact of artificial intelligence in diagnosing premalignant/malignant esophageal and gastric conditions. She is also interested in epidemiology, phenotypes, and the treatment of inflammatory bowel diseases, and she is part of the national and international working groups in this domain. Assoc. Prof. Dr. Daniela Lazar was the author/co-author of several books and book chapters with different gastroenterological, oncological and internal medicine topics for fellows and specialists in these fields, edited by national publishers, and the author of books designated for students. Moreover, Dr. Lazar wrote numerous book chapters and served as the academic editor of several books published by well-known international publishers. Dr. Lazar is also a reviewer for many international journals.

Contents

Preface **IX**

Section 1
Diagnosis and Pathogenesis of Ulcerative Colitis **1**

Chapter 1 **3**
Laboratory Diagnosis of Ulcerative Colitis and the Possibility of Personalized Assessment in Real Conditions
by Gulustan H. Babayeva, Makhir T. Ramazanov, Namig O. Isgandarov and Konul M. Kerimova

Chapter 2 **41**
Non-Invasive Methods of Diagnosis and Management of Patients with Ulcerative Colitis
by Vedran Tomašić, Alen Biščanin, Dominik Kralj, Petra Ćaćić and Doris Ogresta

Chapter 3 **61**
Differential Diagnosis of Ulcerative Colitis
by César Enrique Garnica Camacho

Section 2
Management of Ulcerative Colitis **77**

Chapter 4 **79**
Use of 5-ASA in Ulcerative Colitis in the Era of Biologics
by Ömer Şentürk and Uğur Korkmaz

Chapter 5 **111**
Short- and Long-Term Outcomes of Ileal Pouch Anal Anastomosis versus End Ileostomy after Total Proctocolectomy
by Jonathan Hughes, Sarai Krewson, Griffin Bryant and Bethany Malone

Chapter 6 **125**
Evidence-Based Complementary Therapies for the Management of Ulcerative Colitis
by Vijay Kondreddy, Bhavani Gadiraju and Jhansi Magisetty

Preface

Ulcerative colitis (UC) is a complex, lifelong, immune-mediated inflammatory disorder that affects the rectum and colon to varying degrees, characterized by alternating periods of disease exacerbation and remission. The prevalence of ulcerative colitis was recently estimated to be 5 million cases globally (2023), and the incidence is reported to be increasing worldwide. Pathogenesis is considered multifactorial and not yet fully understood, with both potential genetic and host-related factors implicated in its development. The disease is believed to occur in patients with genetic predisposition following exposure to specific environmental risk factors. Altered microbiota, gut epithelial barrier dysfunction, and dysregulated immune response appear to play a significant role in the pathogenesis of UC.

Clinically, patients present with bloody diarrhea associated with abdominal pain located primarily in the left lower quadrant and fecal urgency. In severe cases, fever and abdominal tenderness may be accompanied by a toxic megacolon. The diagnosis is complex, based on a combination of clinical features and biological, endoscopic and histological aspects. Therefore, the disease alters the quality of life of these patients due to colonic inflammation, leading to the clinical picture represented by chronic diarrhea and rectal bleeding. Moreover, extraintestinal manifestations, including primary sclerosing cholangitis, occur in up to one-third of patients, altering their clinical outcome. The follow-up of these patients is complex, requiring clinical and biological monitoring with a dynamic assessment of inflammatory biomarkers, including fecal calprotectin; also, the longstanding disease is associated with an increased risk of developing colorectal cancer. Therefore, colonoscopic monitoring is recommended starting at 8 years from the UC diagnosis for the surveillance of dysplasia.

The therapeutic management of UC is guided by the patient's risk stratification based on disease location using the Montreal Classification and on disease activity, which may be assessed in clinical practice using several scores, including the Mayo Score.

The goal of pharmacological treatment is initially to induce a rapid clinical, biological, and endoscopic response, and subsequently to maintain both clinical and endoscopic remission. In modern concepts, this also includes achieving histological remission to prevent long-term patient disability. The drugs used for inducing remission include 5-aminosalicylic acid agents and corticosteroids. Maintenance therapy comprises a wide variety of classes of agents, including 5-aminosalicylic acid drugs, thiopurines, biologics such as monoclonal antibodies against tumor necrosis factor, anti-integrins and anti-cytokines, and also the category of small molecules (Janus kinase inhibitors and sphingosine-1-phosphate receptor modulators). The location of the disease and severity of mucosal inflammation determine the selection of drugs and type of delivery. In cases of mild to moderate disease, the first-line treatment for inducing and maintaining remission is represented by 5-aminosalicylic acid. The induction treatment in moderate to severe forms of UC may include oral corticosteroids as a bridge to modern biological treatments used to maintain remission that targets different inflammation pathways. Other experimental and complementary therapeutic approaches, such as fecal microbiota transplantation and probiotic administration, show promising data.

Despite advances in pharmacological approaches to the disease, only one up to two-thirds of the patients will respond to these modern treatments in the context of clinical trials, many of them needing hospitalization and about 7% requiring colectomy in an interval of 5 years after diagnosis. Additionally, the life expectancy of UC patients is shorter than that of the general population. Surgical treatment may be required in case of fulminant or refractory disease. Despite developing novel, potent molecules, approximately 10–20% of patients remain non-responsive and may require proctocolectomy.

This book aims to make an overview of modern concepts referring to the involvement of gut microbiota alteration in the pathogenesis of UC, current laboratory and non-invasive diagnostic assessment of the disease, tips to differentiate UC from other pathologies, including infectious diseases, the role of different classical or complementary therapies and compares the short and long-term outcomes for different surgical type of interventions. Through its updated scientific content and the valuable knowledge offered by authors with extensive experience in this field, the book takes a step forward in understanding this complex disease, a condition that can be extremely challenging for clinicians. It offers guidance for diagnosing and managing ulcerative colitis, enriching readers with a new perspective on the disease.

Nowadays, we own a rich pharmacological arsenal, but the response efficiency is still limited. Therefore, there is an urgent need to improve the management of severe and refractory cases. The key to overcoming therapeutic barriers in the future will likely involve personalized medicine—selecting drugs or drug combinations tailored to individual patients based on their unique phenotypes, as determined by specific tools and biomarkers.

Dr. Daniela Lazăr
Associate Professor,
University of Medicine and Pharmacy "Victor Babeș",
Timișoara, Romania

Section 1

Diagnosis and Pathogenesis of Ulcerative Colitis

Chapter 1

Laboratory Diagnosis of Ulcerative Colitis and the Possibility of Personalized Assessment in Real Conditions

Gulustan H. Babayeva, Makhir T. Ramazanov, Namig O. Isgandarov and Konul M. Kerimova

Abstract

Laboratory diagnostics of ulcerative colitis today are based on a limited number of used laboratory markers; in most cases, these are C-reactive protein and fecal calprotectin. However, given the diversity of ulcerative colitis manifestations, the frequency of relapses and complications, as well as fairly frequent cases of "non-response" to the basic therapy, it is time to reconsider routine views on the laboratory diagnostics of this disease. Taking into account both the features of the clinical course and endoscopic visualization, as well as the constant dependence of diagnostics on pathomorphological assessment, the authors of this chapter offer an extensive review and the results of their own studies related to the use of new laboratory markers for diagnostics and real assessment of the patient's condition without endoscopy and pathomorphology. Only on the basis of a complete assessment of the patient's condition is it possible to build a new personalized approach for further successful therapeutic response in real conditions.

Keywords: ulcerative colitis, fecal markers, "non-response" markers, personification, artificial intelligence

1. Introduction

Ulcerative colitis (UC) is a chronic, relapsing disease that develops due to the interaction of various factors, primarily genetic and environmental factors, and is mainly found in developed countries. The causes of its occurrence are still not precisely established, which complicates treatment and creates the need to improve diagnostic methods. In Europe, there is a geographical gradient vector of incidence "north-west," but despite this, in recent years the frequency of cases has increased in southern and eastern countries. Despite existing treatment methods, patients face severe symptoms and complications, as well as a high risk of disability [1, 2]. There is the concept of undifferentiated colitis, which is used to describe cases where it is impossible to accurately determine whether the disease is ulcerative colitis, Crohn's disease, or other forms of colitis, after analysis of anamnestic and endoscopic data, pathological interpretation of multiple biopsies taken from the colon mucosa and the results appropriate visualization methods [3–10].

Ulcerative colitis can begin at any age [1]. Inflammation usually begins in the rectal area and tends to spread to proximal areas and more than 90% of patients with active UC report the presence of rectal bleeding [11–17].

In addition, with ulcerative proctitis, constipation is also possible; with ulcerative proctosigmoiditis, frequent urge to defecate and tenesmus [12]. The appearance of perianal fistulas should raise suspicion for Crohn's disease (CD).

Unfortunately, with ulcerative proctitis, due to symptoms that appear over several weeks or even months with a tendency to constipation, a sufficient period of time may pass before the patient decides to seek medical help [18].

The onset of severe relapse is observed in approximately 15% of cases, quite often with systemic manifestations, including weight loss, hyperthermia, tachycardia, nausea, vomiting, and manifestations of intoxication [19]. Extraintestinal manifestations, in most cases, are represented by rheumatological lesions (axial, peripheral arthropathy); ophthalmological (episcleritis) and dermatological (erythema nodularis), may occur in 10–20% of cases, and may also precede intestinal symptoms in 10% of patients [20–25].

The ECCO 3E statement [1] states that there is no gold standard for diagnosing ulcerative colitis. Diagnosis is based on clinical, laboratory, imaging, and endoscopic parameters, including histopathology. An infectious cause must be excluded, and if diagnostic doubt remains, a repeat endoscopy with histopathological review may be necessary after some time [EL5].

Laboratory markers have been tested with varying degrees of success. C-reactive phase protein (CRP) has been shown to be less effective in assessing disease activity in UC than in CD, except in cases of acute severe colitis, for which standard values have been established [26, 27]. In patients receiving parenteral steroids, a CRP level greater than 45 mg/L within 48–72 hours of hospitalization for severe colitis with 3–8 bowel movements per day has become an indicator for colectomy [1]. Increased levels of erythrocyte sedimentation rate (ESR), procalcitonin [28], and low albumin levels have also been studied, but have not shown benefits over CRP [1, 2].

The most studied fecal markers are fecal calprotectin and lactoferrin, although other markers such as elastase and S100A12 have also been shown to be accurate in detecting colon inflammation [29, 30].

Calprotectin, determined in feces, correlates well with endoscopic parameters, as well as with relapses and response to therapy, and is therefore useful for diagnosing and assessing the severity of the disease. It can be used as a "relapse marker" in patients with inactive IBD. A doubling of calprotectin levels is associated with an increased risk of relapse (hazard ratio [HR]: 2.01; 95% confidence interval [CI]: 1.52–2.65). However, it is important to note that none of these markers are specific for UC [31].

2. General ideas about laboratory diagnosis of UC

2.1 Use of molecular markers, laboratory diagnostics in a patient with ulcerative colitis at the initial study

The following ECCO 2D statement [1] noted that routine clinical use of genetic or serological molecular markers is not recommended for the classification of ulcerative colitis [EL2] [32–42].

Let us start with an initial examination of laboratory diagnostics in a patient with UC. Initial studies should include a complete blood count, electrolytes, liver and kidney function, iron, vitamin D, C-reactive protein (CRP), and fecal calprotectin [EL5]. You should also check your vaccination status. It is important to exclude infectious diarrhea, including *Clostridium difficile* [EL2] (ECCO Statement 3F) [1, 2].

Laboratory markers of chronic inflammation may remain within normal limits in mild to moderate forms of UC. A complete blood count may show: thrombocytosis—induced by chronic inflammation; anemia is an indicator of severe disease or disease activity; leukocytosis is a predictor of the risk of infectious complications. For ulcerative colitis, with the exception of proctitis, the level of CRP usually corresponds to the severity of the clinical picture [27].

In patients with severe clinical activity of UC, elevated levels of CRP are often accompanied by an increase in ESR, anemia, and hypoalbuminemia. These indicators are used as prognostic biomarkers to assess the need for colectomy in severe acute colitis.

A CRP level greater than 10 mg/L 1 year after the onset of major colitis predicts an increased risk of requiring surgical intervention [1, 43, 44]. CRP levels and ESR are not specific enough to distinguish UC from infectious or other types of colitis. To rule out infectious causes, it is important to perform a stool microbiological examination, including testing for *C. difficile* toxin. Depending on the clinical picture, other tests may be needed, such as testing fresh, warm stool samples for amoebas, protozoa, or parasites to rule out these as possible causes of symptoms. The ECCO 3G document emphasizes that "it is recommended that microbiological testing be performed in patients with recurrent colitis, primarily testing for *C. difficile* and cytomegalovirus [EL3]" [1].

Hospital-acquired *C. difficile* is an increasingly serious public health problem and is associated with higher mortality and increased costs of healthcare resources [45–48]. ECCO recommends screening at every exacerbation of the disease, and stool tests for *C. difficile* testing should be performed whenever treatment resistance or severe relapse occurs [1, 49–51].

Reactivation of cytomegalovirus (CMV) can occur in UC, particularly in immunosuppressed patients with severe relapse [52, 53]. Although CMV reactivation itself may not cause disease relapse and can lead to refractory disease or severe exacerbations. In patients who experience relapses while on immunosuppressive drugs, CMV infection must be ruled out. There is currently no universal method for detecting clinically significant CMV infection in patients with colitis.

However, most experts agree that for diagnosis it is better to use histology and immunohistochemistry of biopsies of the colon mucosa, rather than polymerase chain reaction (PCR) to determine CMV in the blood. Although occasional intranuclear inclusions identified by histopathology as CMV do not necessarily indicate clinically significant infection, the presence of multiple such inclusions usually has greater clinical significance [54–56]. Although there is a laboratory test for CMV avidity, which can help in clinical practice based on percentage detection.

2.2 Biomarkers

Biomarkers are often used for noninvasive monitoring and treatment decision-making in the treatment of patients with UC.

The most widely studied serological markers are perinuclear antineutrophil cytoplasmic antibodies (pANCA) and anti-*Saccharomyces cerevisiae* antibodies

(ASCA). According to various studies, pANCA is found in patients with UC in 65% of cases, and in patients with Crohn's disease in less than 10% of cases [57, 58]. Given the limited sensitivity of the markers, their routine use as the sole means for diagnosing UC and making therapeutic decisions is not justified from a clinical point of view. Various fecal neutrophil proteins (calprotectin, lactoferrin, lysozyme, elastase) have been evaluated as markers of inflammation in IBD [59–62]. But fecal calprotectin appears to be the most sensitive [63].

Numerous studies have repeatedly emphasized the importance of calprotectin in the diagnosis and management of inflammatory bowel diseases (IBD). This marker is useful for:

- Selection of patients for further studies: Calprotectin helps determine which patients require additional diagnostic procedures since its level indicates inflammation.

- Disease severity assessments: Calprotectin values correlate well with inflammatory activity, allowing the severity of the patient's condition to be assessed.

- Detection of disease relapse: An increased level of calprotectin may indicate a relapse, which helps to adjust treatment in time.

- Assessment of treatment effectiveness: A decrease in calprotectin levels indicates a positive effect of therapy and a decrease in the inflammatory process.

Thus, calprotectin is a valuable marker for monitoring IBD and contributes to more accurate decision-making during treatment [31, 64]. But calprotectin does not have the specificity to distinguish between different types of inflammation; however, it represents a useful noninvasive marker in the follow-up of patients with UC [65]. Home calprotectin assessment provides a rapid method for measuring intestinal inflammation, is a reliable alternative to enzyme-linked immunosorbent assay [ELISA], and represents a new way to monitor patients using an online healthcare system [66].

2.3 Examinations upon admission of a patient with acute severe colitis

When a patient is hospitalized with acute severe colitis, a thorough evaluation of complete blood counts, inflammatory markers (CRP or ESR), electrolytes, liver function tests, stool culture, and *C. difficile* toxins should be performed [67].

Predictors of an "unfavorable" outcome:

2.3.1 Anemia

Anemia is common in ulcerative colitis (21% of all patients) [1].

A scheme for estimating total iron requirements is presented in **Table 1**.

The ECCO 5A statement noted that "diagnostic criteria for iron deficiency depend on the level of inflammation. In patients without clinical, endoscopic or biochemical evidence of active disease, a serum ferritin of less than 30 µg/L is an appropriate criterion [EL 2]. In the presence of inflammation, serum ferritin up to 100 µg/L may still be consistent with iron deficiency [EL 4]" [68].

Hemoglobin g/dl	Body weight < 70 kg	Body weight ≥ 70 kg
10–12 [women]	1000 mg	1500 mg
10–13 [men]		
7–10	1500 mg	2000 mg

Table 1.
Simple flowchart for estimating total iron requirements (adapted from Dignass et al. [6]) [68].

Further, the ECCO 5B statement noted that "in the presence of biochemical or clinical signs of inflammation, diagnostic criteria for anemia of chronic disease are serum ferritin greater than 100 μg/L and transferrin saturation less than 20%. If serum ferritin levels are between 30 and 100 μg/L, a combination of true iron deficiency and anemia of chronic disease [EL2] is likely [68].

The most common forms of anemia in UC are iron deficiency anemia, anemia of chronic diseases, as well as their mixtures [69]. Vitamin B12 deficiency, folic acid deficiency, hemolytic anemia, and drug-induced anemia are fewer common forms but should also be considered in the diagnosis [70]. The World Health Organization's definition of anemia is "a decrease in hemoglobin in the blood to a concentration of <12 g/dL [120 g/L] in women and <13 g/dL [130 g/L] in men" [68]. All patients with ulcerative colitis (UC) should undergo screening for anemia, which includes a complete blood count, serum ferritin level, and CRP level measurement.

Tests for anemia include red blood cell distribution width (RDW), mean corpuscular volume (MCV), reticulocyte count, complete blood count, and ferritin and transferrin saturation levels.

Transferrin saturation can decrease in both iron deficiency anemia and inflammation. The level of transferrin receptor in plasma increases with iron deficiency and is not affected by the inflammatory process. If the cause of anemia remains unclear, additional laboratory tests should be performed, including levels of vitamin B12, folate, haptoglobin, and lactate dehydrogenase [6, 68, 71, 72].

2.3.2 Opportunistic infections

The ECCO protocol on opportunistic infections in statement 6A ([4], statement 2B) notes that "patients with ulcerative colitis are at risk of opportunistic infections (taking immunomodulators [EL1], risk higher with combination immunosuppressive therapy [EL3] and patients with malnutrition [EL5]). Concomitant diseases and history of serious infections must be taken into account. Patient age is also an independent risk factor for opportunistic infections in ulcerative colitis [EL3]" [1]. Conditions predisposing to opportunistic infections are classified as severe immunosuppression; human immunodeficiency virus (HIV) infection; limited immunodeficiency [73, 74]. Predisposing factors for opportunistic infections can be both external (e.g., prescribed treatment) and congenital (for example, age, premorbid diseases, malnutrition) [1]. Patients with UC are not immunodeficient themselves but may have altered immune reactivity as a result of their treatment [1]. Older age is an independent risk factor for opportunistic infections and associated adverse events in UC [75]. Corticosteroids increase the risk of opportunistic infections when taken at dosages greater than 20 mg prednisolone per day for more than 2 weeks [76]. All immunosuppressive drugs used in IBD increase the risk of opportunistic infections, and the use of more than one immunosuppressant at the same time can lead to a more than 14-fold increase in risk [1]. This risk is independent of the dose and type of immunosuppressive drug but may depend on the age of the patient [76–78]. Drugs from the group of TNF-α inhibitors double the likelihood of opportunistic infections, in particular tuberculosis [TB] [79].

Among opportunistic infections, special attention throughout the world is paid to the problems of viral hepatitis in this cohort of patients.

Thus, ECCO statement 6B (in Rahier et al. [4], Statement 3B), notes that "all patients with ulcerative colitis should be tested HBsAg, anti-HBAbs, anti-HBcAb at diagnosis for HBV" [1].

The following ECCO 6C statement [4] notes that "after vaccination, the response against HBs should be measured. In patients at risk, the maintenance of antibodies to HBs [EL5] should be monitored [1]. Further, ECCO statement 6E ([4], statement 3E), which states that "reactivation of latent HBV rarely occurs with immunosuppressive therapy used for UC [EL2]. Viremia [HBV DNA] should be assessed every 2–3 months [EL5]" [1].

Patients with UC should also be tested for antibodies to the hepatitis C virus, and if positive, this should be confirmed by positive detection of RNA of this virus. Immunosuppressive therapy alone does not worsen hepatitis C virus infection unless there is co-infection with hepatitis B virus infection or HIV, but it may increase drug-induced hepatotoxicity in patients with hepatitis C virus infection [1].

Given the increased risk of opportunistic infections when immunosuppressive therapy is prescribed, patients with UC should be advised to undergo HIV testing [1]. Seropositivity is not a clear contraindication to immunosuppressive therapy ([4], Statement 3F) [1, 80].

2.3.3 Mycobacterium tuberculosis

I would especially like to touch on the topic of tuberculosis in patients with IBD, so in the ECCO 6F position ([4], position 6A), it is noted that "reactivation of latent tuberculosis in patients treated with anti-TNF increases and is more severe than in the background population [EL2]. Latent tuberculosis should be diagnosed using a combination of patient history, chest X-ray, tuberculin skin test and *interferon-gamma release assays* according to local prevalence and national guidelines. Screening should be considered at diagnosis and always performed before anti-TNF therapy [EL5]. Interferon-gamma release assays are likely complementary to the tuberculin skin test and are preferred for individuals immunized with BCG [EL1]" [1].

2.4 Colorectal cancer and its monitoring in ulcerative colitis

Although it is generally accepted that long-term UC is associated with an increased risk of CRC, reported risk estimates vary widely between studies. Thus, the ECCO 8A statement notes that "the risk of colorectal cancer in ulcerative colitis increases compared with the general population. Risk is associated with disease duration [EL 2], grade [EL 2], and more severe or persistent inflammatory activity [EL 2]." Consistent risk factors for colorectal cancer in ulcerative colitis include: primary sclerosing cholangitis (PSC; with an increased absolute risk of up to 31%) and stable histological activity of the disease [1, 81]. Post-inflammatory polyps may be markers of previous inflammatory severity and have also been identified as a high-risk factor [82]. Family history is also found to be an increased risk, although the risk of this hypothesis varies across studies, as do different claims about gender division (one study found the risk of colorectal cancer to be higher in men (SIR: 2.6; 95% CI: 2.2–3.0) than in women (SIR: 1.9; 95% CI: 1.5–2.3)) [1]. In multivariate logistic regression analysis, colorectal cancer was associated with male gender, disease duration, extensive colitis, concomitant PSC, mean albumin level, and elevated CRP [1].

Today, simple, accessible laboratory tests are used for the early diagnosis of colorectal cancer, in particular, these include fecal TM2-pyruvate kinase and fecal hemoglobin.

3. Fecal markers in laboratory diagnosis of ulcerative colitis

Fecal calprotectin is a protein containing calcium and zinc ions with a molecular weight of 36 kDa. This calcium-containing protein makes up approximately 5% of the total protein and 60% of the cytosolic proteins of neutrophils, that is, neutrophils (the largest group of leukocytes, the main function of which is to protect the body from various infections) are responsible for its production. The protein has bacteriostatic and fungicidal properties; during a gastrointestinal immune response involving neutrophils, calprotectin is released and then excreted in the feces at a concentration six times higher than in the blood. As a result, direct detection of calprotectin in feces clarifies the extent of the inflammatory immune response in the gastrointestinal tract.

The calprotectin test is a noninvasive and inexpensive, but highly sensitive biomarker of intestinal inflammation, which is successfully used in diagnosis, assessing the effectiveness of treatment, predicting relapses, and monitoring the condition of patients with ulcerative colitis and Crohn's disease in remission.

The method makes it possible to distinguish a group of inflammatory diseases from irritable bowel syndrome, in which there is no inflammation of the mucous membrane of the gastrointestinal tract.

The high sensitivity of the calprotectin test has been established and proven for other diseases accompanied by intestinal inflammation: cancer, adenoma, microscopic colitis, intestinal infections with various types of damage to the mucous membrane, including increased permeability and the presence of erosive and ulcerative changes.

The main indications for the calprotectin test are differential diagnosis of organic and functional intestinal diseases; monitoring the activity of inflammation and response to therapy in Crohn's disease, ulcerative colitis; diagnosis of early relapse of chronic IBD; suspicion of intestinal neoplasms (ranks second in importance after the quantitative comprehensive determination of fecal hemoglobin and fecal transferrin); diagnosis of necrotizing enterocolitis in newborns; assessment of the side effects of drugs that damage the intestinal mucosa (enteropathy associated with taking nonsteroidal anti-inflammatory drugs); acute diarrhea syndrome; assessment of the completeness of the inflammatory process, the degree of restoration of the intestinal mucosa after infectious diseases (typhoid fever, escherichiosis, dysentery, viral intestinal infections).

3.1 Fecal lactoferrin

Lactoferrin is a protein from the transferrin family, a globular glycoprotein with a molecular weight of about 80 kDa, widely present in various secretory fluids (milk, saliva, tears, nasal gland secretions). Lactoferrin belongs to the innate immune system; there is evidence that it is indirectly involved in the processes of cellular immunity. The main biological functions of the protein are the binding and transport of iron ions, as well as antibacterial, antiviral, antiparasitic, anticancer, and antiallergic.

Antibacterial activity. The antibacterial properties of lactoferrin are due to its ability to bind iron, which prevents bacterial microflora from using this important microelement for growth and vital activity. However, in addition to this function, lactoferrin also has other mechanisms of anti-infective activity that are not related to iron binding.

Such mechanisms include:

- Stimulation of phagocytosis: Lactoferrin can enhance the process of uptake and destruction of pathogens by phagocytes.

- Effect on complement activity: Lactoferrin may have an effect on the complement system, which helps the body fight infections.

- Specific interaction with bacterial membrane: Lactoferrin can directly interact with the outer membrane of bacteria, leading to their destruction.

In addition, lactoferrin has the ability to destroy bacterial membranes and even penetrate into bacterial cells. The peptide lactoferricin, located at the N-terminus of the lactoferrin molecule, is responsible for specific binding to the bacterial wall. This peptide is released from the lactoferrin molecule upon proteolytic cleavage, for example, using trypsin *in vitro*.

3.1.1 Antivirus activity

Lactoferrin demonstrates antiviral activity against a number of viruses, both human and animal, which may have DNA or RNA genomes. This protein binds to various viral antigens, mainly in laboratory conditions (*in vitro*). Studies have shown its effectiveness against herpes simplex viruses' types 1 and 2, cytomegalovirus, HIV, hepatitis C virus, rotaviruses, poliovirus type 1, adenoviruses, and respiratory syncytial virus. In addition, lactoferrin and its derivative, lactoferricin, inhibit the growth of fungi such as Trichophyton mentagrophytes, which causes skin diseases such as ringworm. Lactoferrin is also effective against *Candida albicans*, a fungus that lives in the oral mucosa of healthy people. The use of lactoferrin as a marker of diarrhea caused by pathogens such as Shigella, Salmonella, Campylobacter, and *Clostridium difficile* is currently being investigated.

This glycoprotein is synthesized by neutrophils, mononuclear phagocytes, and epithelial cells, and is found in secretory fluids such as saliva and breast milk. Its main function is to inhibit bacterial growth and reduce iron availability. The effect of lactoferrin is enhanced by the presence of specific secretory IgA antibodies against bacteria. Under conditions of inflammation in the gastrointestinal tract, neutrophils and phagocytic cells migrate to the inflammatory zone and secrete granules containing lactoferrin. Lactoferrin remains highly stable in feces and can be detected using immunochemical methods. Elevated levels of this biomarker are observed in patients with chronic IBD such as ulcerative colitis and Crohn's disease.

The results of some studies to identify adult patients with IBD showed a "cut-off" level of calprotectin of 50 μg/g of feces; for lactoferrin, a concentration of ≥7.5 μg/g of feces is regarded as positive. The lactoferrin test may be positive in breastfed children and should not be used to evaluate infants (newborns have higher fecal calprotectin levels than older children (median 167 mcg/g)).

Based on the results of a retrospective analysis, fecal lactoferrin may serve as a valuable prognostic biomarker, providing useful information on both long-term treatment outcomes and the risk of colectomy in patients with UC. One published study to evaluate fecal lactoferrin levels as an early predictor of long-term outcomes in UC found interesting results. The study included patients receiving biologics for whom fecal lactoferrin concentration data were available at week 4 of the UNIFI and PURSUIT studies (n = 1063). The evaluation included treatment outcomes such as histological improvement and remission, endoscopic improvement and remission, and clinical remission, each of which was assessed after the completion of the maintenance therapy period. In a subset of the PURSUIT study (n = 667), colectomy cases were recorded from weeks 0 to 228.

Using multivariate logistic analysis and Cox proportional hazards regression analysis, the relationship between fecal lactoferrin levels and treatment outcomes and the likelihood of colectomy was assessed. Elevated levels of fecal lactoferrin at week 4 were found to be associated with adverse long-term outcomes (histological, endoscopic, and clinical). Fecal lactoferrin levels greater than 84.5 μg/mL indicated a decreased likelihood of achieving histological (odds ratio [OR]: 0.27), endoscopic (OR: 0.40), and clinical (OR: 0.43) remission. Notably, the measurement of fecal lactoferrin levels at week 4, along with fecal calprotectin levels and endoscopic and clinical parameters associated with treatment outcomes, provided additional prognostic information. Regarding the risk of colectomy, patients with fecal lactoferrin levels at week 4 ≥ 20.1 and <20.1 μg/mL had colectomy rates of 6.39 and 1.10%, respectively. Patients with fecal lactoferrin levels ≥20.1 μg/mL had a significantly increased risk of colectomy by 99.5% (hazard ratio: 10.95).

Therefore, fecal lactoferrin may serve as a valuable prognostic biomarker for both long-term treatment outcomes and the likelihood of colectomy in patients with ulcerative colitis [83].

3.2 Albumin in feces

Albumin is the main protein in human plasma (40–60%), synthesized by the liver depending on protein intake. The presence of albumin in feces reflects the inflammatory response and intestinal bleeding. Increased levels of albumin and hemoglobin in the stool are found not only in colorectal carcinomas but also in patients with polyps and with Crohn's disease and ulcerative colitis.

Indications for laboratory diagnostics: Establishing the source of bleeding in the lower gastrointestinal tract; diagnosis of colorectal carcinoma; examination of patients at risk; Crohn's disease and ulcerative colitis.

3.3 Eosinophilic neurotoxin (eosinophil-derivedneurotoxin, EDN) in feces

EDN is a cationic glycoprotein that is secreted by activated eosinophils, has strong cytotoxicity, and is of great importance in antiviral defense. It is released from eosinophil granules at sites where eosinophils accumulate at the site where the body meets the pathogen. The accumulation of EDN in the intestine is associated with tissue damage; with its help, it is possible to determine the integrity of the intestinal mucosa in UC and CD, intestinal carcinoma, and intestinal parasitosis. Measurement of eosinophilic neurotoxin in fecal matter can help differentiate between food allergy and food intolerance, as well as assess the effectiveness of an elimination diet. The stool EDN test can serve as an objective parameter of ongoing clinical or subclinical chronic inflammation in the gastrointestinal tract. In patients with ulcerative colitis, EDN allows one to judge the activity and prognosis of the disease.

3.4 β-Defensin-2 in feces

β-Defensins are part of the innate immune system and the antimicrobial immune barrier of the intestinal mucosa. Defensins have antimicrobial activity to varying degrees against some enveloped viruses, bacteria, and fungi. β-defensin-2 deficiency may be observed in the intestinal mucosa of patients with CD. The defensin system in such patients is defective and does not limit invasive bacterial growth, leading to infections typical of CD.

Indication: Differential diagnosis of CD (decreased β-defensin-2 levels) and UC (increased β-defensin levels).

3.5 Hemoglobin-Haptoglobin (Hb-Hp) in fecal

Free hemoglobin (Hb) immediately binds to the serum protein haptoglobin (Hp), forming the Hb-Hp complex, which is more stable in the intestine compared to free hemoglobin. This method can detect bleeding from adenomatous nodes or carcinomas of the upper gastrointestinal tract. The combination of the two analysis methods is highly sensitive and allows for effective detection of colorectal carcinoma in the early stages. Unlike other tests for blood in stool, this method does not require dietary restrictions or special medications. It is capable of detecting free hemoglobin with a sensitivity 100 times greater than that of rapid tests, minimizing the risk of false negative results. Selected antibodies ensure the high specificity of the test, and its results do not depend on the influence of animal hemoglobin, myoglobin, animal and plant peroxidases, or antioxidants. The method is available in enzyme immunoassay and rapid assay formats.

İndications for use: Test for occult blood in stool, Crohn's disease, ulcerative colitis, suspected colon carcinoma, and rectal polyps.

3.6 Fecal myeloperoxidase

Neutrophil granules contain a large number of different enzymes. Myeloperoxidase catalyzes oxidation with the formation of peroxide products toxic to microorganisms. The effectiveness of the bacteria-destroying action is enhanced by the action of polymorphonuclear leukocyte elastase. Determination of myeloperoxidase in feces reflects the activity of Crohn's disease and ulcerative colitis.

Indications: A marker of inflammation of the gastrointestinal tract; oxidative stress.

3.7 Fecal chymotrypsin

Chymotrypsin is a serine protease enzyme that is produced by the pancreas after eating and is involved in the breakdown of food proteins. With insufficiency of pancreatic function, its secretion decreases significantly. Fecal chymotrypsin testing is an informative and noninvasive way to assess pancreatic function. This method measures the concentration of the enzyme, which can be more accurate than assessing its activity. Chymotrypsin remains stable for 12 days at room temperature, making it similar in stability to pancreatic elastase. Therefore, fecal chymotrypsin testing may be an alternative to pancreatic elastase testing. Patients with IBD often have exocrine pancreatic insufficiency.

Indications for chymotrypsin testing: Chronic pancreatitis, exocrine pancreatic insufficiency.

3.8 Fecal pancreatic elastase-1

Elastase-1 is a proteolytic enzyme synthesized exclusively by the pancreas. It is characterized by stability in the intestinal passage and even accumulation: the concentration of elastase is six times higher in feces compared to duodenal juice. Determination of enzyme concentration reflects the secretory capacity of exocrine pancreatic tissue. This method is species-specific and does not cross-react with the porcine enzyme, so patients do not need to interrupt enzyme treatment for testing.

İndication - diagnosis of exocrine pancreatic insufficiency: For chronic pancreatitis; cystic fibrosis; pancreatic carcinoma; insulin-dependent diabetes mellitus; Shwachman-Diamond syndrome; pancreatic insufficiency of another origin (e.g., with UC and CD).

3.9 Fecal lysozyme

Lysozyme (muramidase) is a protein with a molecular weight of about 15 kDa, belonging to the group of alkaline glycosidases. Lysozyme is produced by granulocytes, monocytes, and macrophages. The main source of lysozyme in feces is intestinal granulocytes. It can be detected in the inflammatory infiltrate during the acute period of Crohn's disease. It is also actively secreted by mononuclear cells into the intestinal lumen.

Indications: Diagnosis and monitoring of Crohn's disease; bacterial, viral, allergic and autoimmune IBD.

3.10 Fecal α1-anti-trypsin

α1-Antitrypsin acts as a primary inhibitor of polymorphonuclear neutrophil granulocyte elastase (PMN-elastase) and is secreted during inflammation, reducing the proteolytic activity of PMN-elastase at the site of inflammation, playing an important regulatory role in the anti-inflammatory response.

α1-Antitrypsin is a linear glycoprotein with a molecular weight of 52 kDa, with a free cysteine residue and three side carbohydrate chains. It is synthesized mainly in the liver, as well as by macrophages, monocytes, and epithelial cells of the intestinal mucosa. α1-Antitrypsin is the main inhibitor of serine proteases in human plasma; in addition, fecal α1-antitrypsin is an important marker of intestinal protein loss and increased intestinal permeability, as it is resistant to degradation in the intestine due to its antiproteolytic activity. In addition, measurement of fecal α1-antitrypsin concentrations is used to evaluate and monitor chronic IBD. In clinical practice, assessment of α1-antitrypsin clearance (the ratio of α1-antitrypsin levels in stool to blood) is preferable to a single determination in stool: false negative and false-positive results are reduced by 21%. The method is more sensitive compared to routine methods and facilitates the determination of protein concentration in cell culture supernatants, as well as the successful recognition of both hepatic and intestinal forms of α1-antitrypsin. This method is a promising alternative to the radial immunodiffusion method, especially in cases of large protein loss. The combination of two types of specific antibodies reduces the number of false negative results, ensuring a reliable diagnosis. Thus, this is a new, easy-to-use, and noninvasive test for determining intestinal protein loss.

Indications: Intestinal protein loss syndrome and impaired intestinal permeability; Crohn's disease; complicated ulcerative colitis, necrotizing enterocolitis; inflammation of viral, bacterial, or allergic origin.

3.11 Fecal TM2-pyruvate kinase

Tumor Marker 2 (TM 2) is a dimer of one of the isoforms of the pyruvate kinase enzyme involved in the glycolysis reaction. In normal cells, it is present as a monomer in small quantities, while in tumor cells significant concentrations of the enzyme are produced in the form of a dimer (TM-2). A high concentration of the glycolysis enzyme provides energy expenditure for actively proliferating tumor cells. With the development of precancerous diseases and colon cancer, TM-2 can be detected in stool, which makes it possible to use it as a tumor marker. The "gold standard" for early diagnosis of colon cancer is colonoscopy. However, given its invasiveness and associated risks, it cannot be used as a screening test, unlike the stool TM-2 test, which is a noninvasive method.

The pyruvate kinase test has several advantages over other noninvasive methods. If the presence of heme is detected during a stool occult blood test, this test detects an enzyme specific to tumor cells, which makes it possible to detect both bleeding and non-bleeding neoplasms.

This feature causes a higher sensitivity of the test (for comparison: the sensitivity of the TM-2 test is 92.3%, and the sensitivity of the fecal occult blood test is 20–35%). Unlike the stool occult blood test, the result of this test does not depend on diet and can be obtained with a single collection of biomaterials, which is much more convenient for the patient. In addition, the analysis result is not affected by the use of nonsteroidal anti-inflammatory drugs, vitamin C, gastritis, peptic ulcers, intestinal diverticulosis, and hemorrhoids, that is, false-positive results are practically excluded. A study on TM-2 is indicated for patients with symptoms of colon cancer, as well as with risk factors for its development (smoking, obesity, heredity, age over 50 years, alcohol abuse, sedentary lifestyle, ulcerative colitis). The concentration of TM-2 in feces increases in proportion to tumor growth. Therefore, TM-2 testing can be used to determine the stage and prognosis of the disease. Typically, TM-2 concentrations in feces return to normal after surgery for colon cancer. Receiving a positive test result again or an increase in TM-2 in the postoperative period may indicate a relapse of the disease.

A positive test result suggests the presence of intestinal cancer but does not establish a final diagnosis. To confirm the diagnosis, patients with this result should be referred for additional laboratory and instrumental examinations.

What is the TM2-pyruvate kinase test used for? For early diagnosis of dysplastic polyps and adenocarcinoma of the colon.

When is the study scheduled? If the patient has factors that increase the risk of developing colon cancer: smoking, obesity, heredity, age over 50 years, alcohol abuse, sedentary lifestyle, and ulcerative colitis.

Symptoms of colon cancer: loss of weight and appetite, blood in the stool, iron deficiency anemia (for right-sided tumors), constipation or diarrhea (for left-sided tumors).

4. Hematological markers for laboratory diagnosis of ulcerative colitis

4.1 Homocysteine

The presence of IBD is an independent risk factor for the development of atherosclerosis and, therefore, may be responsible for a high risk of cardiovascular morbidity and mortality [84–86]. Currently, the relationship between hyperhomocysteinemia and the development of thrombosis in IBD has been studied. Hyperhomocysteinemia can be hereditary and also manifests itself with a deficiency of cofactors such as vitamins B6, B1, and folic acid, which are involved in the metabolism of homocysteine.

Homocysteine is a thialactone that forms aggregates with low-density lipoprotein cholesterol, which leads to the formation of foam cells and promotes the reactivation of oxygen-containing radicals. The latter lead to endothelial damage, which in turn causes excessive platelet activation and aggregation.

Reactive oxygen radicals also contribute to the development of thrombosis by oxidizing low-density lipoproteins, which leads to lipid peroxidation, causing the proliferation of vascular smooth muscle. Thus, in studies that examined hyperhomocysteinemia in IBD, it was found that homocysteine levels were significantly higher in people with IBD compared with healthy study participants [83–86]. Our results are also fully consistent with these data [87].

4.2 Antibody studies for laboratory diagnosis of ulcerative colitis

The current concept of the pathogenesis of IBD involves the interaction of individual characteristics of the tolerance of the body's immune system, external factors, and intestinal microflora in genetically predisposed individuals. Only a certain combination of all these factors leads to the development of inflammatory damage to the intestinal mucosa. Many immune-mediated humoral and cellular pathogenetic phenomena have been identified both at the systemic and local (intestinal) levels in IBD. The binding of microbial and food pathogens to Toll- and NOD-like receptors stimulate the activity of macrophages, monocytes, dendritic cells, neutrophils, natural killer cells, innate lymphoid cells, intestinal epithelial cells, inflammasomes and induces the synthesis of proinflammatory cytokines and various tissue factors, which leads to inflammation and destruction of the intestinal wall. Cytokines and tissue antigens enhance autoimmune responses of adaptive immunity, promoting the loss of immunological tolerance and hyperproduction of a wide range of antibodies to both microbial and self-antigens [88].

The search for serological markers of IBD began in 1959, when the first reports of autoantibodies against colonic epithelial cells in UC appeared. Since then, a number of autoantibodies, antimicrobial antibodies, and antibodies to peptide antigens have been identified, including antiglycan antibodies, antineutrophil cytoplasmic antibodies, intestinal goblet cell antibodies, exocrine pancreatic antibodies, and several others, that are associated with CD and UC. Determination of these antibodies makes it possible to identify groups of people at high risk of developing IBD, differentiate CD and UC (especially in cases of undifferentiated colitis), and also individually predict the course of an existing disease, thereby, in some cases, allowing optimization of basic therapy.

4.3 Antineutrophil cytoplasmic antibodies (ANCA)

Antineutrophil cytoplasmic antibodies are a group of autoantibodies against antigens localized in azurophilic and specific granules of neutrophils and monocytes. When ANCA is detected by indirect immunofluorescence (inDIF), depending on the autoantibodies present, several types of neutrophil luminescence are microscopically determined: cytoplasmic (cANCA), perinuclear (pANCA), as well as the so-called atypical luminescence variant or "xANCA." The main antigenic target of cANCA is proteinase 3 (PR3), cANCA is myeloperoxidase (MPO), which are classically highly specific markers of ANCA-associated vasculitis. The atypical fluorescence pattern of ANCA is determined by various antigens of neutrophil granules, including elastase, cathepsin G, lactoferrin, lysozyme, bactericidal permeability-increasing protein (BPI), azurosidine, and is observed in 50% of patients with autoimmune hepatitis, 40% with PSC, 5% with primary biliary cholangitis (PBC), 5–10%—rheumatoid arthritis and IBD [88, 89].

It has been shown that recognition of antigens in the intestinal mucosa is accompanied by local production of ANCA. The mechanism for the appearance of ANCA in IBD may be due to the cross-reactivity of intestinal microflora antigens with human neutrophil antigens. Proteins from the anaerobic bacteria *Bacteroides caccae* (100 kDa) and *Escherichia coli* (OmpC) were identified by Cohavy O. as cross-reactive ANCA epitopes for the colitis-induced T-cell immune response. Most ANCA target antigens play a physiological role in the antimicrobial system of phagocytes. Since ANCA antigens are components of neutrophil granules, their main focus of action is on neutrophil function. It has been shown that ANCA can bind to nuclear antigens of apoptotic neutrophils to form extracellular traps (NETs), the complex of which is a strong immunogenic material and can enhance the inflammatory response in IBD.

For the first time, xANCA of the IgG class in patients with UC was discovered back in 1990 by two independent groups of researchers from the University of California and the University of Freiburg, who reported the occurrence of autoantibodies in 84 and 59% of cases, respectively. In patients with CD, positive titers of xANCA are 10–20% and reach 50–85% among patients with extraintestinal manifestations of IBD in the form of PSC [88–90].

Among the most common and studied xANCA autoantibodies are DNA-lactoferrin complexes, PR3 and cathepsin G. Lactoferrin molecules bound to DNA have high conformational stability, which, when identifying antigenic targets of xANCA, determines the high specificity of the determination of autoantibodies to DNA-lactoferrin complexes. The detection rate of these autoantibodies in patients with UC is 72%, CD—6.3%, PSC—22%, and healthy individuals—2%. Moreover, in half of the patients with PSC, the detection of antibodies to DNA-lactoferrin complexes was associated with the presence of UC in 100% of cases [88–90].

The gold standard for the determination of ANCA is currently the nRIF method on ethanol-fixed neutrophils in combination with determination of the antigenic direction of antibodies—MPO, PR3, cathepsin G, elastase, lactoferrin, lysozyme, bactericidal permeability-increasing protein (BPI) using an enzyme-linked immunosorbent assay, as well as determination of antibodies to the lactoferrin-DNA complex on neutrophils using the nRIF method.

4.3.1 Antibodies to Saccharomyces cerevisiae (ASCA)

The immune response to commensal bacteria is critical to maintaining intestinal mucosal homeostasis, the disruption of which is a key factor in the pathogenesis of IBD. Loss of immunological tolerance to antigens of microbial origin and disruption of intestinal barrier function induce autoimmune responses of adaptive immunity and the production of antibodies directed against bacterial components, thereby maintaining inflammatory damage to the intestinal mucosa in IBD. Examples of such antibodies are anti-glycan antibodies, including anti-*Saccharomyces cerevisiae* (ASCA), anti-mannobioside (AMCA), anti-laminarioside (ALCA), anti-chitobioside (ACCA), anti-laminarin (Anti-L), and anti-chitin antibodies (Anti-C).

Glycans are mono-, oligo-, and polysaccharides that are the predominant surface components of red blood cells, immune cells, and microorganisms, including bacteria and yeast. Possessing structural-modulating properties, glycans are involved in protecting proteins from proteolysis, intercellular interactions, molecular recognition by glycan-binding proteins and maintaining intestinal barrier function.

In 1988, a Scottish study by Main et al. first described the presence of ASCA in patients with CD. The antigenic target of ASCA is a water-soluble thermostable phosphopeptidomannan weighing 200 kDa, the main component of the cell wall of baker's yeast *S. cerevisiae*. Sendid B. and co-authors subsequently found that the epitope for ASCA is phosphopeptidomannan with α-1,3-mannose with n = 1,2-sugar residues [91–94].

Sacharomyces cerevisiae is a yeast commonly used in the food industry for baking and brewing and is probably not directly associated with the pathogenesis of CD. Although the mechanism of ASCA in IBD is still unclear, the mannose-induced immunological response may be due to a cross-reaction with the yeast *Candida albicans*. ASCA has been shown to appear in *Candida albicans*-infected rabbits, but not mice, confirming their potentially cross-reactive nature, which depends on the characteristics of the host organism [91–94]. The induction of ASCA and other antiglycan antibodies has been established in various autoimmune diseases, including IBD, PBC, PSC, and celiac disease. In particular, AMCA, ALCA, and ACCA, despite the fact that their occurrence in patients with CD is no more than 20%, is observed mainly with the onset of the disease at an early age, its complicated course, and the need for surgical treatment. High levels of AMCA and ALCA were combined with the involvement of the small intestine in CD, Anti-L—ileocolitis, Anti-C—penetrating phenotype, and perianal lesions [91–94]. Seropositivity for ACCA and Anti-L was associated with steroid dependence in CD, and the combined detection of ASCA, AMCA, ACCA in concentrations of more than 63 U/ml, 77 U/ml and 50 U/ml, respectively, was associated with a high risk of developing severe exacerbation of CD, with AMCA and ACCA content more than 52 and 25 U/ml, respectively – severe attack of UC [91–94].

The frequency of detection of ASCA classes IgA and/or IgG in patients with CD is 39–70%, UC—10–15%, and in healthy individuals—1–2%. In addition, ASCA occurs in 53% of patients with PSC, 18.9% of PBC, and 55.8% of patients with celiac disease not following a gluten-free diet. An increased detection rate of ASCA has been shown in healthy relatives of patients with CD. Moreover, positive ASCA results were more prevalent in familial rather than sporadic cases of CD. The increased occurrence of ASCA (20–25%) in first-degree relatives of patients with CD is comparable to the role of these antibodies as markers of genetic predisposition. The World Health Organization and ECCO-ESGAR international consensus on the clinical significance of ASCA in IBD allows the use of antibodies to confirm the diagnosis of CD, but not in the differential diagnosis of CD of the colon and UC.

To detect ASCA, the method of enzyme-linked immunosorbent assay (ELISA) is used, less often—indirect immunofluorescence reactions (indirect immunofluorescence reactions) or immunoblotting.

Since the exact structure of the epitopes of antibodies against *S. cerevisiae* has not yet been established, purified and destroyed *S. cerevisiae*, oligopeptidomannans from the cell wall of yeast or mannose are used as a source of antigens in ELISA, which may determine some differences in the interpretation of ASCA detection results [94].

4.4 Diagnostic and prognostic value of ANCA and ASCA

Summarizing the known literature data, it can be confirmed that the indicators of diagnostic sensitivity (DS) and diagnostic specificity (DS) (95% confidence interval, CI) of ASCA in patients with CD vs. UC is 56.6% (51.9–61.3) and 88.1% (85.8–90.0), CD vs. other gastrointestinal diseases (irritable bowel syndrome, diverticulitis, infectious, pseudomembranous and ischemic colitis)—52.8% (44.4–61.1) and 90.9% (77.2–96.7), CD vs. control group (without clinical signs of IBD)—53% (44.6–61.3) and 90.9% (75.6–104.7), respectively. When assessing the diagnostic effectiveness of isolated determination of xANCA in patients with IBD, it was found that the indicators of DC and DC in patients with UC vs. CD vary between 50 and 71% and 75–98%. These data demonstrate that, with limited sensitivity, ASCA and ANCA are highly specific markers of IBD, the use of which is most effective in the differential diagnosis of CD with UC and can serve as an additional confirmatory test in the diagnosis of CD and UC. However, the most interesting is the use of these antibodies in assessing the individual risk of development, and clinical course and predicting complications that require an earlier aggressive treatment strategy for IBD [95, 96].

It was shown that xANCA-positive patients with IBD had a younger age at diagnosis—29.2 ± 11.8 years compared to seronegative patients—43.5 ± 15.3 years [95–97]. It was found that xANCA-seropositive patients with UC had a high likelihood of left-sided intestinal lesions, a severe progressive and often recurrent course. Patients with a diagnostic xANCA titer had a longer duration of disease, frequency of stool, and pyrexia. In addition, thrombocytosis, leukocytosis, and hypoalbuminemia were more common in them. Isolated detection of ANCA with a negative result of ASCA and other antimicrobial antibodies in patients with CD is associated with localization of the lesion in the colon, a UC-like phenotype of CD, and the absence of strictures and penetrations. In UC, high serum levels of ANCA are a predictor of aggressive relapsing disease, the need for early surgical treatment, and the occurrence of pouchitis after the formation of small intestinal pouches [97]. However, other studies have failed to detect clinical differences between xANCA-seropositive and xANCA-seronegative patients with UC and CD.

Of no less interest are the results of studies regarding the relationship between ANCA and predicting response to IBD therapy. It was shown that xANCA-positive patients had a high risk of developing left-sided UC, refractory to 5-ASA, and hormonal therapy, requiring surgical treatment. Negative xANCA status in patients with UC was an independent predictor of early clinical response to infliximab but did not affect the achievement of disease remission [95–97]. However, unlike ANCA-associated vasculitis, autoantibody titers in UC were stable throughout the disease and did not depend on the effectiveness of drug and surgical treatment, which does not allow the use of ANCA detection for monitoring and predicting the inflammatory activity of the disease [98].

According to the results of studies by Schulte-Pelkum and Horn et al., antibodies to PR3 associated with xANCA are a highly specific marker of UC (DS = 58%, DS = 93%). The incidence of PR3-xANCA in patients with UC was 31–39%, CD—1.9–6%, celiac disease—2%, healthy individuals—1.5–2%. High PR3-xANCA titers are directly correlated with severe UC attack according to the Mayo index. It was shown that these antibodies were found in 58.3% of patients with a shorter duration of the disease (0–3 years) compared to patients with a disease duration of 17–20 years (22.7%; $p = 0.0001$), and also significantly more often were determined in patients with total UC (37.3%) vs. left-sided lesions (20.6%, $p = 0.01$) and proctitis (15.4%, $p = 0.04$) [99, 100]. It is important to note that PR3-xANCA was found in 48.1% of patients with a combination of CD and PSC and 40.5% with UC and PSC which allows us to consider the data autoantibodies with an atypical luminescence pattern of ANCA as an unfavorable prognostic marker of extraintestinal manifestations of IBD in the form of PSC [99, 100].

Antibodies against cathepsin G were detected in 40.6% of patients with active UC, and their frequency was significantly higher in patients with severe colitis on endoscopy. In addition, antibodies to cathepsin G were found in 35% of patients with PSC, of whom 80% were diagnosed with IBD. However, some research results demonstrate the lack of correlations of autoantibodies to DNA-lactoferrin complexes, PR3, cathepsin G, BPI, and elastase with clinical signs of IBD [99, 100].

4.4.1 Combined definition of ANCA and ASCA

The diagnosis of CD and UC is based on the results of clinical, radiological, endoscopic, and pathomorphological research methods. In 10–15% of patients, colitis cannot be classified as CD or UC and are considered to have undifferentiated colitis (UC). The diagnosis of NK is usually temporary, and the disease is later finally differentiated into CD or UC. However, in almost 14% of patients, over time, the initial diagnosis of UC changes to CD and vice versa. Accurate and early diagnosis in these cases can be clinically important for making therapeutic decisions and further prognosis. The revised ESPGHAN Porto criteria for IBD in children and adolescents indicate that combined ASCA and xANCA testing may be performed in atypical cases of IBD to differentiate between CD, UC, and unclassified colitis [100]. It follows from this that a comprehensive definition of ASCA and xANCA allows increasing the predictive value of both tests in the diagnosis of CD and UC, especially in cases where the diagnosis cannot be established using traditional clinical and laboratory-instrumental examination methods, and also serves as an informative marker for carrying out differential diagnosis and predicting the characteristics of the clinical course of IBD.

The combined determination of ANCA and ASCA has been evaluated in several studies and has been confirmed as a relevant diagnostic method in UC and CD. Quinton et al. and Peeters et al. found that the combination of ANCA-positive and ASCA-negative results provided 44–57% sensitivity but 97% specificity for UC, while ANCA-negativity combined with ASCA positivity had 49–56% sensitivity and 94–97% specificity for CD [99, 100]. In these studies, the combined use of both tests reduced the DS by approximately 10% but increased the DS to more than 95%, providing a very high predictive value for the diagnosis of UC or CD. A South Korean study found that 49.4% of patients with CD, 61.9% of relatives of patients with CD, and 41.7% of patients with Behçet's disease were ASCA seropositive compared with healthy controls (10%). Seropositivity for ANCA in patients with UC was observed in 44.2% versus 0% of the control group. The combination of a positive ASCA test and a negative ANCA result demonstrated a DR of 48.2% and a DS of -87% for CD, and a combination of a positive ANCA test and a negative ASCA result was 36.4 and 97.6%, respectively, for UC. The authors concluded that both tests can be used in the differential diagnosis of CD and UC, as well as IBD with other colitis accompanied by diarrhea syndrome [99, 100].

A Polish study involving 71 patients with UC, 31 with CD 23 with NC, and 45 functional gastrointestinal disorders showed that the detection rate of ANCA was significantly higher in patients with UC than in CD (68 and 29%, respectively). ASCAs were detected significantly more often in CD (80.6%) than in UC (26.8%). The indicators of PM, DS of positive predictive value (PPV), and negative predictive value (NPV) of ANCA for the diagnosis of UC were 68, 84, 75 and 78%, respectively, ASCA for the diagnosis of CD—81, 78, 45.5 and 95% respectively. The combined use of two markers made it possible to increase the diagnostic accuracy of the test: with a seropositive ANCA result and a negative ASCA in the diagnosis of UC, the values of DC, DS, PCPR, and PCOR were 42, 100, 100 and 43%, respectively, with a negative ANCA result and a positive ASCA in the diagnosis of CD—52, 98.6, 94 and 82%, respectively. Similar results were demonstrated in an Italian study, which showed that ANCAs were detected in 20% of patients with CD versus 50% of patients with UC ($p < 0.05$), while ASCA, on the contrary, were observed in 61% of patients with CD versus 16% patients with UC. The combination of a positive result according to ASCA and a negative result according to ANCA allowed us to obtain such values of DP, DS, and PTPR as 45, 91 and 75%, respectively, in the diagnosis of CD, and the combination of a positive result of ANCA and a negative result of ASCA—44, 95 and 94% respectively in the diagnosis of UC [99, 100].

Thus, ASCA is fundamentally more often detected in patients with CD; on the contrary, pANCA are strictly associated with UC. The limited sensitivity and high specificity of the combined detection of ANCA and ASCA allows the use of these markers in the differential diagnosis of UC and CD and also serves as an additional laboratory examination in the primary diagnosis of IBD.

Whether ANCA and ASCA may be more informative in family and population-based IBD screening needs to be confirmed in prospective studies. As the study of these serological markers continues, it is possible that their use in clinical practice will be more effective in individual long-term prognosis of CD and UC.

5. Diagnosis of celiac disease and lactase deficiency in ulcerative colitis

Celiac disease and ulcerative colitis (UC) are autoimmune intestinal diseases associated with the involvement of tumor necrosis factor-α and interleukin-8 in the pathogenesis [101, 102]. In a study by E. Jandaghi et al., conducted on 406 patients with IBD, the incidence of celiac disease in UC was 1:200, and the levels of serological markers of celiac disease were 10 times higher than in the population [103]. In another study in Italy, among 1711 patients with IBD, 9 (0.5%) patients were diagnosed with celiac disease, established on the basis of serological tests and the results of a morphological study of biopsies of the small intestinal mucosa (SMB). Moreover, these were more often patients with UC and less often—with Crohn's disease [104]. According to Krums et al. [105] of 37 patients with UC and Crohn's disease, an increase in the titer of antibodies to gliadin (AGA) was noted in 8 (21.6%): in 5 (13.5%)—AGA IgA and in 3 (8.1%)—AGA IgG. None of them showed an increase in the level of antibodies to tissue transglutaminase (AtTG). An increase in the level of AGA in patients with IBD may indicate an immunological reaction to gluten and is explained by the increased permeability of SOTC associated with the activity of the inflammatory process [105, 106].

One study aimed to evaluate the risk of developing IBD in patients with celiac disease and vice versa, compared with the general population [107]. The researchers used a histological and general medical registry, which identified 48,551 patients with celiac disease and 83,529 patients with IBD. Patients were matched to individuals from the general population (n = 240,136 were matched to patients with celiac disease and n = 408,195 patients were matched to patients with IBD). Among patients with celiac disease, IBD was diagnosed in 1.6%; in the general population, IBD was diagnosed in 0.4% of patients. Among patients with celiac disease, the risk of developing IBD was almost four times higher (hazard ratio, 3.91 (95% CI 3.56–4.31). The risk of developing Crohn's disease was higher than the risk of developing ulcerative colitis. The incidence of celiac disease was 0.8% among patients with IBD, compared with 0.1% in the general population. The risk of developing celiac disease among patients with IBD was almost 5.5 times higher (hazard ratio, 5.49 [95% CI 4.90–6.16]). The risk of developing celiac disease was higher in patients with ulcerative colitis (seven times higher) than in Crohn's disease (3.3 times higher risk). Typically, the interval between diagnoses was <1 year. During a follow-up period of 20 years, celiac disease was diagnosed in 1.3% of patients with IBD and 2.5% of patients with celiac disease.

To obtain the most complete diagnostic information, the determination of all main serological markers of the disease is used. The study is used to diagnose the disease in case of its mild or atypical course, and can also be used for the purpose of differential diagnosis of celiac disease with other autoimmune diseases of the gastrointestinal tract.

Composition of the study: antibodies to endomysium, IgA; antibodies to tissue transglutaminase, IgG; antibodies to tissue transglutaminase, IgA; total immunoglobulin A (IgA) in serum; antibodies to deaminated gliadin peptides, IgA; antibodies to deaminated gliadin peptides, IgG. To detect autoantibodies in celiac disease, two main methods are used: indirect immunofluorescence reaction (IRIF) and enzyme-linked immunosorbent assay (ELISA).

Using RNIF, autoantibodies to gliadin are detected. They interact with one of the main components of gluten (gliadin). These tests are quite sensitive, but not very specific. Thus, antibodies to gliadin can be detected not only in celiac disease but also in autoimmune hepatitis, systemic lupus erythematosus, rheumatoid arthritis, and other autoimmune diseases.

Using ELISA, autoantibodies to endomysium and tissue transglutaminase can be detected. Antibodies to endomysium are autoantibodies that interact with the connective tissue sheath of the muscle fiber (endomysium). Antibodies to tissue transglutaminase interact with the enzyme involved in the biochemical transformations of gliadin. These studies are characterized by very high sensitivity and specificity. Thus, antibodies to tissue transglutaminase, IgA, are considered the best clinical and laboratory marker of celiac disease.

Total IgA antibodies are an important factor in the local protection of mucous membranes. They bind to microorganisms and prevent their penetration from external surfaces deep into tissues, enhancing the phagocytosis of antigens by activating complement along the alternative pathway. IgA deficiency is often associated with autoimmune pathologies—enteropathies accompanied by protein loss.

A comprehensive study of the entire spectrum of autoimmune antibodies allows us to obtain the most complete information about the patient. A complete serological test is performed to diagnose celiac disease in patients with symptoms of this disease. With celiac disease, the following symptoms may be observed: chronic diarrhea or constipation, weight loss, iron deficiency anemia, unmotivated fatigue, and others (identical for UC and CD). It should be noted that now the atypical and erased form of celiac disease is more often observed. For this reason, a complete laboratory examination is also carried out on all patients at risk for this disease, regardless of whether they have symptoms of the disease or not. The risk group for celiac disease includes patients with the following diseases: type 1 diabetes mellitus, isolated deficiency of immunoglobulin IgA, autoimmune thyroid diseases, Down syndrome, Turner syndrome, Williams syndrome, autoimmune liver diseases, as well as first-degree relatives of patients with celiac disease.

Positive result (antibodies to deaminated gliadin peptides): celiac disease; rheumatoid arthritis; systemic lupus erythematosus; sarcoidosis; Sjögren's syndrome; IgA nephropathy; autoimmune hepatitis; primary biliary cirrhosis; irritable bowel syndrome.

A positive result (endomysium antibodies, tissue transglutaminase antibodies): celiac disease.

A negative result (for all antibody variants): absence of celiac disease; disease control on the background of a gluten-free diet.

A negative result (antibodies to endomysium, IgA, antibodies to gliadin, IgA, antibodies to tissue transglutaminase, IgA): isolated (selective) deficiency of immunoglobulins of the IgA class.

What can influence the result? Prescribing a gluten-free diet before taking blood for testing may lead to a false negative result [108, 109].

Lactase deficiency is a condition associated with decreased activity of the lactase enzyme. Lactase is produced by cells of the small intestine - enterocytes. Its function is to break down lactose (milk sugar) entering the intestines into glucose and galactose. Lactose is the only carbohydrate in breast milk and the first sugar that enters the newborn's body. In addition to breast milk, lactose is found in animal milk and dairy products. When there is a deficiency of the lactase enzyme in the body, a clinical syndrome develops, characterizing the inability to digest and absorb lactose - this condition is called "lactose intolerance." The incidence of lactase deficiency varies greatly by population. If among the peoples of northwestern Europe, about 1–3% of adults cannot digest lactose, then among the indigenous populations of Africa, Asia, and Latin America their number is close to 90–100%.

There is primary lactase deficiency, in which intestinal cells (enterocytes) are not changed, and secondary lactase deficiency, when a decrease in enzyme activity is associated specifically with damage to enterocytes.

5.1 Diagnosis of lactase deficiency

Typically, the diagnosis is made based on the presence of symptoms characteristic of lactase deficiency and the patient's positive response to treatment. However, for an accurate diagnosis, a genetic test is performed to detect lactase deficiency. Lactase deficiency is caused by decreased transcription of the LCT gene encoding the enzyme. In close proximity to the LCT gene is the MCM6 gene, which influences the expression pattern of the lactase gene. It has been proven that the replacement of cytosine (C) with thymine (T) in the 13th intron of the MCM6 gene increases the expression of the lactase gene. Carriers of the main allele C are characterized by a decrease in lactase levels in adulthood, that is, lactase deficiency. Carriers of the minor T allele, on the contrary, can digest lactose, and this ability is not lost over time.

Information about the genotype based on the C (−13,910) T marker of the MSM6 gene will help the doctor choose the right low-lactose or no-lactose diet for adult patients, prevent digestive disorders in children, and assess the risk of developing osteoporosis in women during menopause.

Interpretation of MCM6 results (C(−13,910)T).

C/C is a genotype associated with lactose intolerance in adults.

C/T is a genotype associated with good lactose tolerance in adults.

T/T is a genotype associated with good lactose tolerance in adults.

The results of the study should be interpreted by a doctor in conjunction with other genetic, anamnestic, clinical, and laboratory data on IBD.

6. Determination of the interleukin series in ulcerative colitis

According to modern views, the development of ulcerative colitis (UC) is based on genetically determined disturbances in the interaction of receptors of the innate immune system and the molecular structures of microorganisms (PAMPs, pathogen-associated molecular patterns), loss of immunological tolerance in relation to autologous microflora, pathogenic activation of the innate and adaptive immune systems, accompanied by hyperproduction of various inflammatory factors, including the system of proinflammatory cytokines [110–112]. Traditionally, the immunopathogenesis of UC is associated with dysregulation of Th2 cell and NKT cell populations. However, the accumulation of data on new proinflammatory cell populations (Th17) and cytokines (IL-17, IL-33), the duality of functions of individual cytokines (TGF-β), overestimation of the anti-inflammatory and underestimation of the proinflammatory functions of other cytokines lead to a revision of some positions, including substantiate the role of Th1 (IFN-γ) cells and Th17 (IL-17) cells and associated proinflammatory cytokines (TNF-α - tumor necrosis factor-α, IL-1β, IL-6, IL-17) in immunopathogenesis not only Crohn's disease, but also UC [113, 114].

The presented data show that IL-8, as well as the following IL-1β, IL-6, and TNF-α in terms of production, constitute the main cytokine profile of the operated colon with pronounced inflammatory activity in combination with a severe clinical course associated with resistance to drug therapy. IL-1β is produced mainly by cells of the innate immune system (monocytes, macrophages, etc.) and, according to the results of many studies, is a pluripotent proinflammatory cytokine [115]. It causes activation and degranulation of granulocytes and macrophages with the release of oxygen radicals, nitric oxide, prostaglandins, leukotrienes, proteases, and other factors of inflammation and destruction. The spread and intensification of inflammation are facilitated by the effects of IL-1β, associated with an increase in the permeability of endothelial and epithelial cells, activation of cytotoxic T cells, as well as stimulation of the secretion of chemotactic cytokines, including IL-8, which persists for a long time at the site of inflammation, being the main highly selective chemoattractant of neutrophils during IBD. Its level in colon tissue correlates with the number of neutrophils, the presence of which in the cellular infiltrate is a sign of active UC [115].

The cytokines IL-6 and especially TNF-α, which is the main target of anti-cytokine therapy, also have high proinflammatory activity. IL-6 regulates the acute phase of inflammation by stimulating the production of acute-phase proteins and the recycling of macrophages, monocytes, and lymphocytes through the activation of chemokines and adhesion molecules [116].

TNF-α, like IL-1β, enhances the proinflammatory functions of neutrophils and macrophages; among its many effects, activation of Th1 cells and stimulation of IL-8 secretion are also highlighted. An increase in the content of IFN-γ in colon biopsies is associated with the activation of Th1 and NK cells and is realized in increased intracellular lysis of pathogens in macrophages, differentiation of Th1 cells, and activation of B cells [116, 117]. The presence of IL-17 in biopsies reflects the function of Th17 cells, which are involved in the pathogenesis of many inflammatory diseases, including experimental colitis. According to the results of most studies, an increase in the number of Th1 and Th17 cells and the level of their corresponding IFN-γ and IL-17 is associated with the pathogenesis of CD [117, 118]. Therefore, an increase in the concentration of these cytokines in the colon of patients with UC indicates the presence of common cross-talk mechanisms with CD. At the same time, the absence of IL-4 and IL-5 cytokines in biopsy specimens does not confirm the pathogenic role of Th2 cells at the final (destructive) stage of uncontrolled inflammation [119].

7. The role of eosinophilic inflammation and features of its laboratory diagnosis in ulcerative colitis

Data on the role of eosinophils in the formation and progression of fibrotic changes, as well as the development and maintenance of inflammatory processes in patients with UC and CD, are limited. Eosinophils have been recognized as important players in immune cell infiltration in IBD, including eosinophilic infiltration into the lamina propria, as reflected in the Geboes histological index for UC [120, 121]. One of the predictors of lack of therapeutic response is the presence of eosinophilic infiltration in the lamina propria in biopsies of the mucous membrane in patients with UC [122]. The high content of mediators in eosinophil granules involved in inflammation and/or fibrosis makes these cells particularly interesting in the context of fibrostenosis in IBD and in the search for new "targets" for treatment [123].

7.1 Eosinophil cationic protein (ECP)

Degranulation of eosinophils releases eosinophil-specific ECP, also known as ribonuclease-3, which is a protein with a molecular weight of 18–22 kDa. ECP has the ability to damage cell membranes by forming pores in transmembrane channels through which toxic molecules can enter the cell. Eosinophils contain large amounts of ECP, which is released upon degranulation, and therefore de novo synthesis is not required during degranulation [120].

Patients with active UC and CD had increased serum EPC levels compared with healthy controls or patients with IBD in remission [124, 125].

7.2 Eosinophil peroxidase (EPO)

Toxic cationic EPO produces hypohalous, bromous, and hypochlorous acids by utilizing hydrogen peroxide, halide ions, and bromide through the formation of these acids. EPO can cause cell damage [126]. Biopsies from the colon mucosa of patients with CD and perfusion fluids from the colon of patients with UC show increased levels of EPO at the time of relapse [127].

7.3 Eosinophil-derived neurotoxin (EDN)

Contrary to its name, EDN is not neurotoxic to the human body (neuropathological reactions were detected in a mouse model) [127]. Amcoff K. and his co-authors reported increased levels of EDN protein in the feces of patients with UC not only at the time of relapse but also 3 months before relapse. Therefore, fecal EDN has been proposed as a biomarker or predictor of relapse [128, 129]. Thus, EDN may serve as a diagnostic tool or biomarker for gastrointestinal inflammation. Whether this protein additionally contributes to direct inflammation or fibrosis is still a matter of debate.

7.4 Eosinophil basic protein (MBP)

MBP, proteoglycan 2 (PRG2), is encoded by the PRG2 gene and is represented by MBP1 (can be found in eosinophils, basophils, and mast cells) and MBP2 (present only in eosinophils). Due to its cationic nature, this protein can disrupt the permeability and functioning of cell membranes. It is believed that MBP, due to its toxicity, directly increases the permeability of the epithelial layer [130].

8. Possibilities for personalizing laboratory diagnostics of ulcerative colitis

The diagnosis of IBD is established based on generally accepted criteria in accordance with the recommendations of the European Crohn's and Colitis Organization, the American gastro-associations, the World gastro-association, etc., based in general on old and new/modified indices, including isolated endoscopic indices, combined indices taking into account the general condition of the patient, endoscopic, clinical and laboratory parameters. Unfortunately, in most cases, for a full assessment within such indices, a time period is sometimes required for the full compliance of aspects of the assessment within one or another index.

At the same time, laboratory diagnostics, based mainly on taking into account only two parameters (CRP and calprotectin), in our opinion, need to be expanded and modernized.

With all this in mind, we made an attempt to create a system for assessing the patient's condition on the basis of other laboratory studies.

The aim of the study: To create a monitoring system for the condition of patients with IBD.

Materials and methods: In the period from August 2015 to June 2022, 388 patients with a diagnosis of IBD. The diagnosis was established on the basis of generally accepted criteria in accordance with the recommendations of the European Crohn's and Colitis Organization. The severity of the clinical course of the disease is assessed in accordance with the Truelove-Witts Index and Mayo in the case of UC and Crohn's Disease Activity Index and Harvey-Bradshaw index in CD. The study did not include patients with severe cardiac and nephrological pathology, as well as those who underwent surgery within the last 6 months or are in the stage of clinical and endoscopic remission. Thus, the study included 250 patients; of these, 112 (44.8%) had CD and 138 (55.2%) UC. The age of patients was from 18 to 60 years (39.4 ± 4.6), by gender: 129 (51.6%) women and 121 (48.4%) men. The duration of the disease before contacting a specialist doctor was 1.1–8.3 years (3.7 ± 1.2), and patients were under dynamic observation from 6 to 48 months (18.4 ± 7.2). In addition to the general clinical examination, the following laboratory markers were obligatory determined: highly sensitive C-reactive protein (h/s-CRP), homocysteine, vitamin D, platelet level, ECP, α-TNF, IL-1β, IL-2, IL-4, IL-6, IL-8, IL-10, IL-18 in blood, calprotectin, lactoferrin and TM-2-pyruvate kinase (TM2-P) in feces, albumin level (micro- and macro) in urine. Patients, if necessary, underwent repeated studies (680 cases in total). In the statistical processing of the results obtained, the generally accepted methods of descriptive statistics were used with the calculation of the arithmetic mean values of the trait (M), standard deviation (σ), and mean error (m). Student's coefficient t was used when comparing quantitative values in groups; the error probability (p) was determined. To establish the relationship between the indicators, the Pearson correlation coefficient ® was calculated.

Results of the study and their discussion: Separate analysis of the detection of each of these indicators in the UC and CD groups did not reveal any difference ($p > 0.05$). There was also no difference when analyzing the results by gender ($p > 0.05$).

We carried out computer processing of the obtained data in order to find a possible relationship between the indicators of endothelial dysfunction and the condition of patients, determined in accordance with the recommendations. The severity of changes in the studied indicators of endothelial dysfunction was assessed as a percentage of the permissible value of the norm (with an increase in the indicator, its excess of the upper limit of the norm, and a decrease compared to the lower limit, with a reduced content). The results obtained are presented in **Table 2**.

Laboratory indicator/ severity	Norm	I degree (mild)	II degree (medium-severe)	III degree (severe)
h/s CRP	N	1,3 N	1,5 N	>1,5 N
Homocysteine	N	1,3 N	1,5 N	>1,5 N
Platelets	N	1,1 N	1,2 N	>1,2 N
Vitamin D	N	0,7 N	0,4 N	<0,4 N
Eosinophilic cationic protein	N	1,1 N	1,2 N	>1,2 N
Fecal calprotectin	N	2 N	3 N	>3 N
Albumin in urine	N	—	Micro-	Macro-
Points	0	1	2	3

Table 2.
Correlation of some indicators of endothelial dysfunction, inflammation, and the severity of the clinical course in patients with inflammatory bowel disease.

As a result, it was found that if there is a severity of endothelial dysfunction, estimated from 4 to 6 points, patients with IBD have a mild, from 6 to 9 points—medium, and if there is more than nine points—a high degree of severity of the clinical course of the disease. Clinical and endoscopic remission corresponded to three points or less. The degree of correlation was 0.863.

Separately, the correlations of some fecal markers and the severity of the clinical course in patients with IBD were studied, and the results are presented in **Table 3** as an index for calculating the activity of the disease.

Interpretation: 0 points—no severity (clinical and endoscopic remission)

From 0.1 to 3 points—mild severity.

From 3 to 6 points—moderate severity

From 6 to 9 points—severe degree

Above 9 points—very high degree of activity

The possible correlation of some laboratory parameters was also studied (in patients with a tendency to strictures (stenoses) and concomitant infectious processes (latent tuberculosis, herpes viruses), the results are presented in **Table 4** as a new calculation index.

Laboratory indicator/ severity	Norm	I degree (mild)	II degree (moderate)	III degree (severe)	IV degree (super severe)
Fecal calprotectin	N	Less 2 N	From 2 to 3 N	From 3 to 5 N	More 5 N
Fecal lactoferrin	N	Less 2 N	From 2 to 3 N	From 3 to 4 N	More 4 N
Fecal TM2-pyruvatikine	N	Less 1.5 N	From 1.5 to 2.5 N	From 2.5 to 5 N	More 5 N
Points	0	1	2	3	

Table 3.
Correlation of some fecal indicators and the severity of the clinical course in patients with inflammatory bowel diseases.

Laboratory indicator/ severity	Norm	I degree (mild)	II degree (moderate)	III degree (severe)	IV degree (super severe)
h/s CRP	N	1.5 N	2 N	3 N	4 N
Eosinophilic cationic protein	N	1.2 N	1.5 N	2 N	3 N
Vitamin D	N	0.7 N	0.5 N	0.3 N	0.2 N
IL-8	N	1.2 N	1.4 N	1.6 N	1.8 N
IL-18	N	1.2 N	1.4 N	1.6 N	1.8 N
Fecal calprotectin	N	Less 2 N	From 2 to 3 N	From 3 to 5 N	More 5 N
Fecal lactoferrin	N	Less 2 N	From 2 to 3 N	From 3 to 4 N	More 4 N
Fecal TM2-pyruvatikine	N	Less 1.5 N	From 1.5 to 2.5 N	From 2.5 to 5 N	More 5 N
Points	0	1	2	3	

Table 4.
Correlation of some indicators and the severity of the clinical course in patients with inflammatory bowel diseases, noted in patients with a concomitant infectious process and the presence of strictures.

Interpretation: 0 points—no severity (clinical and endoscopic remission)
From 0.1 to 3 points—mild severity.
From 3 to 6 points—moderate severity
From 6 to 9 points—severe degree
Above 9 points—very high degree of activity.

With the help of machine learning artificial intelligence, threshold values were derived for some indicators that predict relapse in patients with IBD, here are some of them: an increase in h/s CRP above 1.2 mg/L, homocysteine higher than 7.4 μmol/L, platelets above 328,000/mm^3, a decrease in the level of vitamin D below 45.6 ng/mL, an increase in the level of fecal calprotectin above 88 μg/g and albumin in the urine above 6 mg/L.

We have selected the most accessible, both in practical (availability/availability in the laboratory network) and in economic terms, studies of indicators of endothelial dysfunction and immuno-allergic changes. These indicators were: homocysteine, platelets, highly sensitive CRP, ECP, and vitamin D in the blood, fecal calprotectin, lactoferrin, and TM2-P, as well as microalbumin in the urine [87, 131].

Our results allow us to conclude that the severity of some indicators of endothelial dysfunction, as well as immuno-allergic changes, directly correlates with the severity of the patient's condition.

The expanded laboratory diagnostics of UC that we have proposed allows, with the diagnosis established, not to resort to repeated expensive studies and to obtain real-time results that enable a personalized assessment of the severity of the patient's condition. This allows creating an individual system for monitoring the patient's condition, making timely decisions about the need for additional studies, and adjusting therapy, which is especially important in outpatient practice.

9. Conclusion

As presented above, ulcerative colitis is a chronic relapsing disease characterized not only by serious intestinal complications but also by a large number of extraintestinal complications. Questions of "no answer" to the therapy being carried out are in most cases hidden in the depths of laboratory diagnostics. So, for example, for this group of patients, in matters of hormonal resistance or hormonal dependence, it is necessary to study the laboratory parameters of the steroid-adrenal panel. One can cite many "crisis" scenarios with the only hope for the "light at the end of the tunnel," which includes laboratory diagnostics with its growing capabilities in the modern world. Approaching the issue of laboratory diagnosis of this pathology based on the determination of a small number of studies (as stated above, mainly CRP, fecal calprotectin) is currently incorrect. It is necessary to maintain a personalized approach in the laboratory diagnosis of ulcerative colitis, which will help in the early identification of many aggravating factors in the future treatment of this pathology. As they say, "if you are forewarned, you are already forearmed."

Conflict of interest

The authors declare no conflict of interest.

Author details

Gulustan H. Babayeva[1]*, Makhir T. Ramazanov[2], Namig O. Isgandarov[3] and Konul M. Kerimova[4]

1 Azerbaijan State Advanced Training Institute for Doctors named after A. Aliyev, Department of Therapy, Baku, Azerbaijan

2 Memorial Hospital, Chief Physician of the Laboratory Department, Baku, Azerbaijan

3 Memorial Hospital, Head of the Laboratory, Baku, Azerbaijan

4 Science Research Institute of Lung Diseases, Baku, Azerbaijan

*Address all correspondence to: ghbabayeva@gmail.com

References

[1] Magro F, Gionchetti P, Eliakim R, Ardizzone S, Armuzzi A, et al. Third European evidence-based consensus on diagnosis and management of ulcerative colitis. Part 1: Definitions, diagnosis, extra-intestinal manifestations, pregnancy, cancer surveillance, surgery, and ileo-anal pouch disorders. Journal of Crohn's and Colitis. 2017;**2**:649-670. DOI: 10.1093/ecco-jcc/jjx008

[2] Lozoya Angulo ME, de Las Heras Gómez I, Martinez Villanueva M, et al. Faecal calprotectin, a useful marker in discriminating between inflammatory bowel disease and functional gastrointestinal disorders. Gastroenterología y Hepatología. 2017;**40**:125-131

[3] Mirkov MU, Verstockt B, Cleynen I. Genetics of inflammatory bowel disease: Beyond NOD2. The Lancet Gastroenterology & Hepatology. 2017;**2**:224-234

[4] Rahier JF, Magro F, Abreu C, et al. Second European evidence-based consensus on the prevention, diagnosis and management of opportunistic infections in inflammatory bowel disease. Journal of Crohn's & Colitis. 2014;**8**:443-468

[5] Testa A, Rispo A, Romano M, et al. The burden of anaemia in patients with inflammatory bowel diseases. Digestive and Liver Disease. 2016;**48**:267-270

[6] Dignass AU, Gasche C, Bettenworth D, et al. European consensus on the diagnosis and management of iron deficiency and anaemia in inflammatory bowel diseases. Journal of Crohn's & Colitis. 2015;**9**:211-222

[7] Goodhand JR, Kamperidis N, Rao A, et al. Prevalence and management of anemia in children, adolescents, and adults with inflammatory bowel disease. Inflammatory Bowel Diseases. 2012;**18**:513-519

[8] Martin J, Radeke HH, Dignass A, Stein J. Current evaluation and management of anemia in patients with inflammatory bowel disease. Expert Review of Gastroenterology & Hepatology. 2017;**11**:19-32

[9] Adler SN, Yoav M, Eitan S, Yehuda C, Eliakim R. Does capsule endoscopy have an added value in patients with perianal disease and a negative work up for Crohn's disease? World Journal of Gastrointestinal Endoscopy. 2012;**4**:185-188

[10] Gionchetti P, Dignass A, Danese S, et al. Third European evidence-based consensus on the diagnosis and management of Crohn's disease 2016. Part 2: Surgical management and special situations. Journal of Crohn's & Colitis. 2017;**11**:135-149

[11] Shah SC, Colombel JF, Sands BE, Narula N. Mucosal healing is associated with improved long-term outcomes of patients with ulcerative colitis: A systematic review and meta-analysis. Clinical Gastroenterology and Hepatology. 2016;**14**:1245-55.e8

[12] Peyrin-Biroulet L, Sandborn W, Sands BE, et al. Selecting therapeutic targets in inflammatory bowel disease [STRIDE]: Determining therapeutic goals for treat-to-target. The American Journal of Gastroenterology. 2015;**110**:1324-1338

[13] Cholapranee A, Hazlewood GS, Kaplan GG, Peyrin-Biroulet L,

Ananthakrishnan AN. Systematic review with meta-analysis: Comparative efficacy of biologics for induction and maintenance of mucosal healing in Crohn's disease and ulcerative colitis controlled trials. Alimentary Pharmacology & Therapeutics. 2017;**45**:1291-1302

[14] Mosli MH, Zou G, Garg SK, et al. C-reactive protein, fecal calprotectin, and stool lactoferrin for detection of endoscopic activity in symptomatic inflammatory bowel disease patients: A systematic review and meta-analysis. The American Journal of Gastroenterology. 2015;**110**:802-819; quiz 820

[15] Zittan E, Kelly OB, Kirsch R, et al. Low fecal calprotectin correlates with histological remission and mucosal healing in ulcerative colitis and colonic Crohn's disease. Inflammatory Bowel Diseases. 2016;**22**:623-630

[16] Lee SH, Kim MJ, Chang K, et al. Fecal calprotectin predicts complete mucosal healing and better correlates with the ulcerative colitis endoscopic index of severity than with the Mayo endoscopic subscore in patients with ulcerative colitis. BMC Gastroenterology. 2017;**17**:110

[17] Patel A, Panchal H. Dubinsky MC Fecal calprotectin levels predict histological healing in ulcerative colitis. Inflammatory Bowel Diseases. 2017;**23**:1600-1604

[18] Parente F, Molteni M, Marino B, et al. Are colonoscopy and bowel ultrasound useful for assessing response to short-term therapy and predicting disease outcome of moderate-to-severe forms of ulcerative colitis? A prospective study. The American Journal of Gastroenterology. 2010;**105**:1150-1157

[19] Yamamoto T, Shimoyama T, Matsumoto K. Consecutive monitoring of faecal calprotectin during mesalazine suppository therapy for active rectal inflammation in ulcerative colitis. Alimentary Pharmacology & Therapeutics. 2015;**42**:549-558

[20] Ellrichmann M, Wietzke-Braun P, Dhar S, et al. Endoscopic ultrasound of the colon for the differentiation of Crohn's disease and ulcerative colitis in comparison with healthy controls. Alimentary Pharmacology & Therapeutics. 2014;**39**:823-833

[21] Colombel JF, Rutgeerts PJ, Sandborn WJ, et al. Adalimumab induces deep remission in patients with Crohn's disease. Clinical Gastroenterology and Hepatology. 2014;**12**:414-22.e5

[22] Colombel JF, Reinisch W, Mantzaris GJ, et al. Randomised clinical trial: Deep remission in biologic and immunomodulator naïve patients with Crohn's disease a SONIC post hoc analysis. Alimentary Pharmacology & Therapeutics. 2015;**41**:734-746

[23] Carvalho PB, Rosa B, Cotter J. Mucosal healing in Crohn's disease are we reaching as far as possible with capsule endoscopy? Journal of Crohn's & Colitis. 2014;**8**:1566-1567

[24] Peyrin-Biroulet L, Reinisch W, Colombel JF, et al. Clinical disease activity, C-reactive protein normalisation and mucosal healing in Crohn's disease in the SONIC trial. Gut. 2014;**63**:88-95

[25] Kucharzik T, Wittig BM, Helwig U, et al. Use of intestinal ultrasound to monitor Crohn's disease activity. Clinical Gastroenterology and Hepatology. 2017;**15**:535-42.e2

[26] Kopylov U, Yablecovitch D, Lahat A, et al. Detection of small bowel mucosal healing and deep remission in patients with known small bowel Crohn's disease

using biomarkers, capsule endoscopy, and imaging. The American Journal of Gastroenterology. 2015;**110**:1316-1323

[27] Kopylov U, Yung DE, Engel T, et al. Fecal calprotectin for the prediction of small bowel Crohn's disease by capsule endoscopy: A systematic review and meta-analysis. European Journal of Gastroenterology & Hepatology. 2016;**28**:1137-1144

[28] Van Weyenberg SJ, Bouman K, Jacobs MA, et al. Comparison of MR enteroclysis with video capsule endoscopy in the investigation of small-intestinal disease. Abdominal Imaging. 2013;**38**:42-51

[29] Höög CM, Bark LÅ, Arkani J, Gorsetman J, Broström O, Sjöqvist U. Capsule retentions and incomplete capsule endoscopy examinations: An analysis of 2300 examinations. Gastroenterology Research and Practice. 2012;**2012**:518718

[30] Nemeth A, Kopylov U, Koulaouzidis A, et al. Use of patency capsule in patients with established Crohn's disease. Endoscopy. 2016;**48**:373-379

[31] Jensen MD, Brodersen JB, Kjeldsen J. Capsule endoscopy for the diagnosis and follow up of Crohn's disease: A comprehensive review of current status. Annals of Gastroenterology. 2017;**30**:168-178

[32] Samuel S, Bruining DH, Loftus EV Jr, et al. Endoscopic skipping of the distal terminal ileum in Crohn's disease can lead to negative results from ileocolonoscopy. Clinical Gastroenterology and Hepatology. 2012;**10**:1253-1259

[33] Qiu Y, Mao R, Chen BL, et al. Systematic review with meta-analysis: Magnetic resonance enterography vs. computed tomography enterography for evaluating disease activity in small bowel Crohn's disease. Alimentary Pharmacology & Therapeutics. 2014;**40**:134-146

[34] Puylaert CA, Tielbeek JA, Bipat S, Stoker J. Grading of Crohn's disease activity using CT, MRI, US and scintigraphy: A meta-analysis. European Radiology. 2015;**25**:3295-3313

[35] Mendoza JL, González-Lama Y, Taxonera C, et al. Using of magnetic resonance enterography in the management of Crohn's disease of the small intestine: First year of experience. Revista Española de Enfermedades Digestivas. 2012;**104**:578-583

[36] Castiglione F, Mainenti PP, De Palma GD, et al. Noninvasive diagnosis of small bowel Crohn's disease: Direct comparison of bowel sonography and magnetic resonance enterography. Inflammatory Bowel Diseases. 2013;**19**:991-998

[37] Taylor SA, Mallett S, Bhatnagar G, et al. Diagnostic accuracy of magnetic resonance enterography and small bowel ultrasound for the extent and activity of newly diagnosed and relapsed Crohn's disease [METRIC]: A multicentre trial. The Lancet Gastroenterology & Hepatology. 2018;**3**:548-558

[38] Calabrese E, Maaser C, Zorzi F, et al. Bowel ultrasonography in the management of Crohn's disease. A review with recommendations of an international panel of experts. Inflammatory Bowel Diseases. 2016;**22**:1168-1183

[39] Choi M, Lim S, Choi MG, Shim KN, Lee SH. Effectiveness of capsule endoscopy compared with other diagnostic modalities in patients with small bowel Crohn's disease:

A meta-analysis. Gut and Liver. 2017;**11**:62-72

[40] Monteiro S, Dias de Castro F, Boal Carvalho P, et al. Essential role of small bowel capsule endoscopy in reclassification of colonic inflammatory bowel disease type unclassified. World. Journal of Gastrointestinal Endoscopy. 2017;**9**:34-40

[41] Panes J, Bouhnik Y, Reinisch W, et al. Imaging techniques for assessment of inflammatory bowel disease: Joint ECCO and ESGAR evidence-based consensus guidelines. Journal of Crohn's & Colitis. 2013;**7**:556-585

[42] Siddiqui MR, Ashrafian H, Tozer P, et al. A diagnostic accuracy meta-analysis of endoanal ultrasound and MRI for perianal fistula assessment. Diseases of the Colon and Rectum. 2012;**55**:576-585

[43] Gecse KB, Bemelman W, Kamm MA, et al. A global consensus on the classification, diagnosis and multidisciplinary treatment of perianal fistulising Crohn's disease. Gut. 2014;**63**:1381-1392

[44] Yanai H, Lichtenstein L, Assa A, et al. Levels of drug and antidrug antibodies are associated with outcome of interventions after loss of response to infliximab or adalimumab. Clinical Gastroenterology and Hepatology. 2015;**13**:522-30.e2

[45] Ordás I, Mould DR, Feagan BG, Sandborn WJ. Anti-TNF monoclonal antibodies in inflammatory bowel disease: Pharmacokinetics-based dosing paradigms. Clinical Pharmacology and Therapeutics. 2012;**91**:635-646

[46] Vande Casteele N, Khanna R, Levesque BG, et al. The relationship between infliximab concentrations, antibodies to infliximab and disease activity in Crohn's disease. Gut. 2015;**64**:1539-1545

[47] Moore C, Corbett G, Moss AC. Systematic review and meta-analysis: Serum infliximab levels during maintenance therapy and outcomes in inflammatory bowel disease. Journal of Crohn's & Colitis. 2016;**10**:619-625

[48] Langhorst J, Boone J, Lauche R, Rueffer A, Dobos G. Faecal lactoferrin, calprotectin, PMN-elastase, CRP, and white blood cell count as indicators for mucosal healing and clinical course of disease in patients with mild to moderate ulcerative colitis: Post hoc analysis of a prospective clinical trial. Journal of Crohn's & Colitis. 2016;**10**:786-794

[49] Alomair A, Alswayeh A, Alhazmi A, Alshammari A, Alsaffar S, et al. Intestinal inflammation markers in inflammatory bowel disease. International Journal of Community Medicine and Public Health. 2018;**5**(3):829-833. DOI: 10.18203/2394-6040.ijcmph20180401

[50] Harzallah I, Rigaill J, Williet N, Paul S, Roblin X. Golimumab pharmacokinetics in ulcerative colitis: A literature review. Therapeutic Advances in Gastroenterology. 2017;**10**:89-100

[51] Vande Casteele N, Ferrante M, Van Assche G, et al. Trough concentrations of infliximab guide dosing for patients with inflammatory bowel disease. Gastroenterology. 2015;**148**:1320-9.e3

[52] Zittan E, Kabakchiev B, Milgrom R, et al. Higher adalimumab drug levels are associated with mucosal healing in patients with Crohn's disease. Journal of Crohn's & Colitis. 2016;**10**:510-515

[53] Brandse JF, van den Brink GR, Wildenberg ME, et al. Loss of infliximab into feces is associated

with lack of response to therapy in patients with severe ulcerative colitis. Gastroenterology. 2015;**149**:350-5.e2

[54] Heida A, Park KT, van Rheenen PF. Clinical utility of fecal calprotectin monitoring in asymptomatic patients with inflammatory bowel disease: A systematic review and practical guide. Inflammatory Bowel Diseases. 2017;**23**:894-902

[55] Yamamoto T, Shimoyama T, Umegae S, Matsumoto K. Serial monitoring of faecal calprotectin for the assessment of endoscopic recurrence in asymptomatic patients after ileocolonic resection for Crohn's disease: A long-term prospective study. Therapeutic Advances in Gastroenterology. 2016;**9**:664-670

[56] Zhulina Y, Cao Y, Amcoff K, Carlson M, Tysk C, Halfvarson J. The prognostic significance of faecal calprotectin in patients with inactive inflammatory bowel disease. Alimentary Pharmacology & Therapeutics. 2016;**44**:495-504

[57] Ferreiro-Iglesias R, Barreiro-de Acosta M, Otero Santiago M, et al. Fecal calprotectin as predictor of relapse in patients with inflammatory bowel disease under maintenance infliximab therapy. Journal of Clinical Gastroenterology. 2016;**50**:147-151

[58] De Vos M, Dewit O, D'Haens G, et al. Fast and sharp decrease in calprotectin predicts remission by infliximab in anti-TNF naïve patients with ulcerative colitis. Journal of Crohn's & Colitis. 2012;**6**:557-562

[59] Mao R, Xiao YL, Gao X, et al. Fecal calprotectin in predicting relapse of inflammatory bowel diseases: A meta-analysis of prospective studies. Inflammatory Bowel Diseases. 2012;**18**:1894-1899

[60] Theede K, Holck S, Ibsen P, Kallemose T, Nordgaard-Lassen I, Nielsen AM. Fecal calprotectin predicts relapse and histological mucosal healing in ulcerative colitis. Inflammatory Bowel Diseases. 2016;**22**:1042-1048

[61] Lasson A, Öhman L, Stotzer PO, et al. Pharmacological intervention based on fecal calprotectin levels in patients with ulcerative colitis at high risk of a relapse: A prospective, randomized, controlled study. United European Gastroenterology Journal. 2015;**3**:72-79

[62] De Vos M, Louis EJ, Jahnsen J, et al. Consecutive fecal calprotectin measurements to predict relapse in patients with ulcerative colitis receiving infliximab maintenance therapy. Inflammatory Bowel Diseases. 2013;**19**:2111-2117

[63] Diederen K, Hoekman DR, Leek A, et al. Raised faecal calprotectin is associated with subsequent symptomatic relapse, in children and adolescents with inflammatory bowel disease in clinical remission. Alimentary Pharmacology & Therapeutics. 2017;**45**:951-960

[64] Du L et al. Within-stool and within-day sample variability of fecal calprotectin in patients with inflammatory bowel disease: A prospective observational study. Journal of Clinical Gastroenterology. 2018;**52**:235-240

[65] Colombel JF, Panaccione R, Bossuyt P, et al. Effect of tight control management on Crohn's disease [CALM]: A multicentre, randomised, controlled phase 3 trial. Lancet. 2018;**390**:2779-2789

[66] van Rheenen P. Do not read single calprotectin measurements in isolation when monitoring your patients with inflammatory bowel disease. Inflammatory Bowel Diseases. 2014;**20**:1416-1417

[67] Negrón ME, Rezaie A, Barkema HW, et al. Ulcerative colitis patients with clostridium difficile are at increased risk of death, colectomy, and postoperative complications: A population-based inception cohort study. The American Journal of Gastroenterology. 2016;**111**:691-704

[68] Vinding KK, Elsberg H, Thorkilgaard T, et al. Fecal calprotectin measured by patients at home using smartphones–a new clinical tool in monitoring patients with inflammatory bowel disease. Inflammatory Bowel Diseases. 2016;**22**:336-344

[69] Greenup AJ, Bressler B, Rosenfeld G. Medical imaging in small bowel Crohn's disease-computer tomography enterography, magnetic resonance enterography, and ultrasound: "Which one is the best for what?". Inflammatory Bowel Diseases. 2016;**22**:1246-1261

[70] Pellino G, Nicolai E, Catalano OA, et al. PET/MR versus PET/CT imaging: Impact on the clinical management of small bowel Crohn's disease. Journal of Crohn's & Colitis. 2016;**10**:277-285

[71] Schoepfer AM, Beglinger C, Straumann A, et al. Fecal calprotectin more accurately reflects endoscopic activity of ulcerative colitis than the Lichtiger Index, C-reactive protein, platelets, hemoglobin, and blood leukocytes. Inflammatory Bowel Diseases. 2013;**19**:332-341

[72] Jang HJ, Choi MH, Eun CS, et al. Clinical usefulness of double balloon enteroscopy in suspected Crohn's disease: The KASID multi-center trial. Hepato-Gastroenterology. 2014;**61**:1292-1296

[73] Bettenworth D, Gustaversusson A, Atreja A, et al. A pooled analysis of efficacy, safety, and long-term outcome of endoscopic balloon dilation therapy for patients with stricturing Crohn's disease. Inflammatory Bowel Diseases. 2017;**23**:133-142

[74] Jess T, Rungoe C, Peyrin-Biroulet L. Risk of colorectal cancer in patients with ulcerative colitis: A meta-analysis of population-based cohort studies. Clinical Gastroenterology and Hepatology. 2012;**10**:639-645

[75] Eaden JA, Abrams KR, Mayberry JF. The risk of colorectal cancer in ulcerative colitis: A meta-analysis. Gut. 2001;**48**:526-535

[76] Lovasz BD, Lakatos L, Golovics PA, et al. Risk of colorectal cancer in Crohn's disease patients with colonic involvement and stenosing disease in a population-based cohort from Hungary. Journal of Gastrointestinal and Liver Diseases. 2013;**22**:265-268

[77] Fumery M, Pineton de Chambrun G, Stefanescu C, et al. Detection of dysplasia or cancer in 3.5% of patients with inflammatory bowel disease and colonic strictures. Clinical Gastroenterology and Hepatology. 2015;**13**:1770-1775

[78] Rieder F, Latella G, Magro F, et al. European Crohn's and colitis organisation topical review on prediction, diagnosis and management of fibrostenosing Crohn's disease. Journal of Crohn's & Colitis. 2016;**10**:873-885

[79] Ripollés T, Martínez-Pérez MJ, Paredes JM, Vizuete J, García-Martínez E, Jiménez-Restrepo DH. Contrast-enhanced ultrasound in the differentiation between phlegmon and abscess in Crohn's disease and other abdominal conditions. European Journal of Radiology. 2013;**82**:e525-e531

[80] Martínez MJ, Ripollés T, Paredes JM, Blanc E, Martí-Bonmatí L. Assessment of the extension and the inflammatory

activity in Crohn's disease: Comparison of ultrasound and MRI. Abdominal Imaging. 2009;**34**:141-148

[81] Magro F, Langner C, Driessen A, et al. European consensus on the histopathology of inflammatory bowel disease. Journal of Crohn's & Colitis. 2013;7:827-851

[82] Li XH et al. Diffusion-weighted MRI enables to accurately grade inflammatory activity in patients of ileocolonic Crohn's disease: Results from an observational study. Inflammatory Bowel Diseases. 2017;**23**:244-253

[83] Chen R et al. Fecal lactoferrin early predicts long-term outcomes in ulcerative colitis: A post-hoc analysis of the UNIFI and PURSUIT trials. United European Gastroenterology Journal. Jul 2023;**11**(6):542-550. DOI: 10.1002/ueg2.12431 Available from: https://europepmc.org/article/med/37350349

[84] Alkan E, Serkan M, Yildirim B. Atherosclerosis in inflammatory bowel disease. The Turkish Journal of Gastroenterology. 2014;**25**(1):20-25. DOI: 10.5152/tjg.2014.4443

[85] Oldenburg B, Fijnheer R, Griend R. Homocysteine in inflammatory bowel disease: A risk factor for thromboembolic complications. The American Journal of Gastroenterology. 2000;**95**:2825-2830. DOI: 10.1111/j.1572-0241.2000.03193.x

[86] Romagnuolo J, Fedorak R, Dias V. Hyperhomocysteinemia and inflammatory bowel disease: Prevalence and predictors in a cross-sectional study. The American Journal of Gastroenterology. 2001;**96**:2143-2149. DOI: 10.1111/j.1572-0241.2001.03950.x

[87] Babayeva GH, Babayev ZM. Frequency of detection of some markers of endothelial dysfunction in patients with inflammatory bowel diseases. ТЕРАПЕВТИЧЕСКИЙ АРХИВ. 2018;**4**:12-16. DOI: 10.26442/terarkh201890412-16

[88] Padoan A, Musso G, Contran N, Basso D. Inflammation, autoinflammation and autoimmunity in inflammatory bowel diseases. Current Issues in Molecular Biology. 2023;**45**(7):5534-5557. DOI: 10.3390/cimb45070350

[89] Kuznetsova DA, Lapin SV, Shchukina OB. The diagnostic and prognostic value of serological markers of inflammatory bowel diseases (a literature review). Almanac of Clinical Medicine. 2020;**48**(6):364-374. DOI: 10.18786/2072-0505-2020-48-061

[90] Nuij VJ, Zelinkova Z, Rijk MC, Beukers R, Ouwendijk RJ, Quispel R, et al. Phenotype of inflammatory bowel disease at diagnosis in the Netherlands: A population-based inception cohort study (the Delta Cohort). Inflammatory Bowel Diseases. 2013;**19**(10):2215-2222. DOI: 10.1097/MIB.0b013e3182961626

[91] Lerner A. Autoantibody profile in inflammatory bowel disease. In: Shoenfeld Y, Meroni PL, Gershwin ME, editors. Autoantibodies. 3rd ed. Elsevier; 2014. pp. 419-424

[92] Mitsuyama K, Niwa M, Takedatsu H, Yamasaki H, Kuwaki K, et al. Antibody markers in the diagnosis of inflammatory bowel disease. World Journal of Gastroenterology. 2016;**22**(3):1304-1310. DOI: 10.3748/wjg.v22.i3.1304

[93] Baum LG, Cobb BA. The direct and indirect effects of glycans on immune function. Glycobiology. 2017;**27**(7):619-624. DOI: 10.1093/glycob/cwx036

[94] Conrad K, Schößler W, Hiepe F, Fritzler MJ. Autoantibodies in Organ

Specific Autoimmune Diseases – A Diagnostic Reference: Autoantigens, Autoantibodies, Autoimmunity. 2nd ed. Pabst: Wolfgang Science; 2017

[95] Pang Y, Ruan H, Wu D, Lang Y, Sun K, Xu C. Assessment of clinical activity and severity using serum ANCA and ASCA antibodies in patients with ulcerative colitis. Allergy, Asthma and Clinical Immunology. 2020;**16**:37. DOI: 10.1186/s13223-020-00433-1

[96] Zhou G, Song Y, Yang W, Guo Y, Fang L, Chen Y, et al. ASCA, ANCA, ALCA and many more: Are they useful in the diagnosis of inflammatory bowel disease? Digestive Diseases. 2016;**34**(1-2):90-97. DOI: 10.1159/000442934

[97] Lee WI, Subramaniam K, Hawkins CA, Randall KL. The significance of ANCA positivity in patients with inflammatory bowel disease. Pathology. 2019;**51**(6):634-639. DOI: 10.1016/j.pathol.2019.07.002

[98] Александрова ЕН, Новиков АА, Лукина ГВ, Парфенов АИ. Клиническое значение антител при воспалительных заболеваниях кишечника. Therapeutic Archive. 2021;**93**(2):228-235. DOI: 10.26442/00403660.2021.02.200610

[99] Moiseev S, Cohen Tervaert JW, Arimura Y, et al. 2020 international consensus on ANCA testing beyond systemic vasculitis. Autoimmunity Reviews. 2020;**19**(9):102618. DOI: 10.1016/j.autrev.2020. 102618

[100] Levine A, Koletzko S, Turner D, et al. ESPGHAN revised porto criteria for the diagnosis of inflammatory bowel disease in children and adolescents. Journal of Pediatric Gastroenterology and Nutrition. 2014;**58**(6):795-806. DOI: 10.1097/MPG.0000000000000239

[101] Paskual V, Dieli-Crimi R, Lopez-Palacios N, Bodas A, Medrano L, Nunez C. Inflammatory bowel disease and celiac disease: Overlaps and differences. World Journal of Gastroenterology. 2014;**20**(17):4846-4856. DOI: 10.3748/wig.20i17.4846

[102] Kocsis D, Toth Z, Csontos AA, Miheller P, Pak P, et al. Prevalence of inflammatory bowel disease among celiac disease patients in a Hungarian celiac Centre. BMC Gastroenterology. 2015;**15**:141. DOI: 10.1186/s12876-015-0370-7

[103] Jandaghi E, Hojatnia M, Vahedi H, Shahbaz-Khani B. Is the prevalence of celiac disease higher than general population in inflammatory bowel disease? Middle East Journal of Digestive Diseases. 2015;7(2):82-87

[104] Casella G, Di Bella C, Salemme M, Villanacci V, Antonelli E, Baldini V, et al. Celiac disease. Non-celiac gluten sensitivity and inflammatory bowel disease. Minerva Gastroenterologica e Dietologica. 2015;**61**(4):267-271

[105] Krums LM, Babaian AF, Bykova SV, et al. Celiac disease associated with ulcerative colitis. Therapeutic Archive. 2019;**91**(2):87-90. DOI: 10.26442/00403660.2019.02.000152

[106] Bykova SV, Sabelnikova EA, Gudkova PB, Drozdov VN, Shcherbakov PL, et al. Celiac disease rate in gastroenterological patients. Therapeutic Archive. 2016;**88**(2):39-43. (In Russ.). DOI: 01716/terarkh201688239-43

[107] Karl M, Jonas S, Benjamin L, et al. Association of celiac disease and inflammatory bowel disease: A nationwide register-based cohort study. The American

Journal of Gastroenterology. 1 Sep 2022;**117**(9):1471-1481. DOI: 10.14309/ajg.0000000000001834

[108] Armstrong D, Don-Wauchope AC, Verdu EF. Testing for gluten-related disorders in clinical practice: The role of serology in managing the spectrum of gluten sensitivity. Canadian Journal of Gastroenterology. 2011;**25**(4):193-197

[109] Nandiwada SL, Tebo AE. Testing for antireticulin antibodies in patients with celiac disease is obsolete: A review of recommendations for serologic screening and the literature. Clinical and Vaccine Immunology. 2013;**20**(4):447-451. DOI: 10.1128/CVI.00568-12

[110] Konovich EA, Shirokikh KYe, Khalif IL, Shapina MV. Colonic cytokines for severe ulcerative colitis. Ros Zhurn Gastroenterol Hepatol Coloproctol. 2016;**42**(1):93-98

[111] Konovich EA, Khalif IL, Shapina MV. Immunopathogenesis of inflammatory bowel diseases. Ros Zhurn Gastroenterol Hepatol Coloproctol. 2013;**23**(4):69-77

[112] Fiocci C. Etiopathogenesis of inflammatory bowel disease. Coloproctology. 2015;**1**:5-20

[113] Biancheri P, Di Sabatino A, Ammoscato F, et al. Absence of a role for interleukin-13 in inflammatory bowel disease. European Journal of Immunology. 2014;**44**:370-385

[114] Pushparaj P, Li D, Komai-Koma M, et al. Interleukin-33 exacerbates acute colitis via interleukin-4 in mice. Immunology. 2013;**140**:70-77

[115] MacDonald TT, Monteleone G. Adaptive immunity: Effector and inhibitory cytokine pathways in gut inflammation. In: Targan SR, Shanahan F, Karp LC, editors. Inflammatory Bowel Disease. Translating Basic Science into Clinical Practice. Chichester: Wiley-Blackwell; 2010. pp. 82-91

[116] Mudter J, Neurath MF. IL-6 signaling in inflammatory bowel disease: Pathophysiological role and clinical relevance. Inflammatory Bowel Diseases. 2007;**13**:1016-1023

[117] Maillard MH, Snapper SB. Cytokines and chemokines in mucosal homeostasis. In: Targan SR, Shanahan F, Karp LC, editors. Inflammatory Bowel Disease. Translating Basic Science into Clinical Practice. Chichester: WileyBlackwell; 2010. pp. 119-156

[118] Strober W, Fuss IJ. Proinflammatory cytokines in the pathogenesis of inflammatory bowel diseases. Gastroenterology. 2011;**140**(6):1756-1767

[119] Műzes G, Molnar B, Tulassay Z, Sipos F. Changes of the cytokine profile in inflammatory bowel diseases. World Journal of Gastroenterology. 2012;**18**(41):5848-5861

[120] Jacobs I, Ceulemans M, Wauters L, Breynaert C, Vermeire S, Verstockt B, et al. Role of eosinophils in intestinal inflammation and fibrosis in inflammatory bowel disease: An overlooked villain? Frontiers in Immunology. 2021;**12**:754413. DOI: 10.3389/fimmu.2021.754413

[121] Canavese G, Villanacci V, Antonelli E, Cadei M, Sapino A, Rocca R, et al. Eosinophilia – Associated basal plasmacytosis: An early and sensitive histologic feature of inflammatory bowel disease. APMIS. 2017;**125**:179-183. DOI: 10.1111/apm.12639

[122] Zezos P, Patsiaoura K, Nakos A, Mpoumponaris A, Vassiliadis T, Giouleme O, et al. Severe eosinophilic

infiltration in colonic biopsies predicts patients with ulcerative colitis not responding to medical therapy. Colorectal Disease. 2014;**16**:O420-O430. DOI: 10.1111/codi.12725

[123] Shah K, Ignacio A, McCoy KD, Harris NL. The emerging roles of eosinophils in mucosal homeostasis. Mucosal Immunology. 2020;**13**:574-583. DOI: 10.1038/s41385-020-0281-y

[124] Wędrychowicz A, Tomasik P, Pieczarkowski S, Grzenda-Adamek Z, Kowalska-Duplaga K, Fyderek K. Clinical value of serum eosinophilic cationic protein assessment in children with inflammatory bowel disease. Archives of Medical Science. 2014;**10**:1142-1146. DOI: 10.5114/aoms.2013.34415

[125] Abedin N, Seemann T, Kleinfeld S, Ruehrup J, Röseler S, Trautwein C, et al. Fecal eosinophil cationic protein is a diagnostic and predictive biomarker in young adults with inflammatory bowel disease. Journal of Clinical Medicine. 2019;**8**:2025. DOI: 10.3390/jcm8122025

[126] Kovalszki A, Weller PF. Chapter 24: Eosinophils and eosinophilia. In: Rich R, Fleisher T, Shearer W, Schroeder H, Frew A, Weyand C, editors. Clinical Immunology. London: Elsevier; 2013. pp. 349-361

[127] Woodruff SA, Masterson JC, Fillon S, Robinson ZD, Furuta GT. Role of eosinophils in inflammatory bowel and gastrointestinal diseases. Journal of Pediatric Gastroenterology and Nutrition. 2011;**52**:650-661. DOI: 10.1097/MPG.0b013e3182128512

[128] Amcoff K, Cao Y, Zhulina Y, Lampinen M, Halfvarson J, Carlson M. Prognostic significance of faecal eosinophil granule proteins in inflammatory bowel disease. Scandinavian Journal of Gastroenterology. 2019;**54**:1237-1244. DOI: 10.1080/00365521.2019.1670251

[129] Roca M, Varela AR, Donat E, Cano F, Hervas D, Armisen A, et al. Fecal calprotectin and eosinophil-derived neurotoxin in healthy children between 0 and 12 years. Journal of Pediatric Gastroenterology and Nutrition. 2017;**65**:394-398. DOI: 10.1097/MPG.0000000000001542

[130] Plager DA, Loegering DA, Checkel JL, Tang J, Kephart GM, Caffes PL, et al. Major basic protein homolog (MBP2): A specific human eosinophil marker. Journal of Immunology. 2006;**177**:7340-7345. DOI: 10.4049/jimmunol.177.10.7340

[131] Babayeva GH, Babayev ZM. New approach to the estimation of a clinical flow in patients with ulcerative colitis and Crohn's disease. Experimental and Clinical Gastroenterology. 2019;**162**(2):19-23. (In Russ.). DOI: 10.31146/1682-8658-ecg-162-2-19-23

Chapter 2

Non-Invasive Methods of Diagnosis and Management of Patients with Ulcerative Colitis

Vedran Tomašić, Alen Biščanin, Dominik Kralj, Petra Ćaćić and Doris Ogresta

Abstract

The global incidence and age-standardized prevalence rate of ulcerative colitis (UC) is increasing worldwide. It is a debilitating and lifelong inflammatory disease affecting both pediatric and adult patients. Thus, it is important to focus on modern treat-to-target approach, based on a tight control of the disease with close monitoring through interval assessments and modification of the treatment. Endoscopy remains the key method for UC assessment, but recent guidelines focus on implementation of non-invasive methods for UC diagnosis and management such as biomarkers (C-reactive protein, fecal calprotectin, and fecal lactofferin) and imaging methods (intestinal ultrasound). We summarize the diagnostic performance of non-invasive tests and present current evidence-based non-invasive strategy recommendations for UC monitoring.

Keywords: ulcerative colitis, non-invasive monitoring, biomarkers, CRP, fecal calprotectin, fecal lactoferrin, intestinal ultrasound

1. Introduction

Given the chronicity, relapsing-remitting course (with structural damage, extraintestinal manifestations, bowel surgery, and colorectal dysplasia/neoplasia/carcinogenesis), impact of the disease (symptom burden, negative impact on the quality of life [QoL], fatigue, anxiety-depressive disorder [ADD], and disability), and the treatment-related complications on the ulcerative colitis (UC) patients, it comes as no surprise that contemporary management algorithms and consensus guidelines are complex and ever-changing. Rapid advent and incorporation of widely available novel diagnostic tools continues discussions on "best" new goals and targets based on available data. For practicing inflammatory bowel disease (IBD) specialists, there are practical and demanding realities in translating limitations of current one-size-fits-all guidelines to real life and clinical practice. These clinicians are burdened with the knowledge that, despite constant advances, gaining the optimal and satisfactory outcome is achievable in some (and certainly not most) UC patients. The traditional goals of treating UC are physical and psychological symptoms resolution with normalization of QoL and avoidance of restorative proctocolectomy [1]. This is challenged by the fact that major unmet needs such as sustained long-term steroid-free remission, histologic-endoscopic mucosal remission, and bowel urgency remission are the ones that are causally linked with improved long-term outcomes (such as prevention of progression to "damage" or "carcinogenesis"). Therefore, regulatory agencies incorporate objective outcomes, such as endoscopy and histology, with co-primary endpoints of symptom assessment such as patient-reported outcomes (PROs) in trial designs. Insurers covering the cost of UC diagnosis and management follow that practice. But UC is lifelong disease with the need for frequent and longitudinal serial assessment of disease activity with multiple objective tools. A "treat-to-target" (T2T) strategy based on serial measurements of activity and severity of disease and response to treatment with close monitoring of intestinal inflammation are the recommended contemporary approaches to UC [2]. Frequent endoscopic assessment is considered "gold standard" for UC disease monitoring and management by multiple international guidelines [3–5]. Although proactive endoscopic assessment of bowel inflammation is associated with improved long-term outcomes, there are multiple differences in its utilization [6]. Given the invasive nature and high cost of frequent and repeated endoscopies needed to monitor UC, search for non-invasive diagnostic alternatives is warranted. In the first systematic review (10 studies evaluating 1846 participants) of patient perceptions of monitoring tools in IBD, adult IBD patients preferred non-invasive investigations (such as fecal calprotectin [FC] and intestinal ultrasound [IUS]) [7]. Recent evidence-based American Gastroenterological Association (AGA) guidelines propose non-invasive biomarkers as a first-line strategy for monitoring UC patients which can inform treatment decisions and avoid unnecessary routine endoscopic assessment of disease [8].

2. Non-invasive methods for diagnosis and management of UC patients

2.1 Clinical activity indices/scoring systems

Interval symptom-based monitoring strategy is still valid and often used, especially in the group of asymptomatic UC patients who place high value on avoiding biomarkers collecting and/or testing [8]. The potential benefit of symptom-based monitoring is the ease of collecting PROs; potential disadvantages are higher risk of developing disease complications (risk of relapse, structural damage, and dysplasia). This does not suggest that symptom resolution is unimportant; it is an elementary but insufficient long-term treatment target. Various clinical activity and scoring systems are still used as a means of evaluating the severity of UC. Truelove-Witts Score consists of six variables (number of stools, fever, tachycardia, hemoglobin level, erythrocyte sedimentation rate [ESR]/C-reactive protein [CRP], and weight loss/gain) and has been the basis of severity index scoring in UC, although with several limitations (unclear definitions of improvement and/or worsening, focus on disease activity during a single moment) [9]. Since Trulove and Witts study, multiple scores have been developed to describe disease severity. Mayo Score is most widely used scoring system in clinical trials as well as in routine practice [10]. It consists of four components: stool frequency (SF), rectal bleeding (RB), findings of endoscopy, and physician's global assessment (ranging 0–12; three points for each component).

There are several disadvantages of Mayo score. It incorporates endoscopic assessment with all the burden that invasive tests place on UC patients. Some of its endoscopic variables have been reported to have significant interobserver variability (namely mucosal friability). And clearly, there is the subjectivity of the physical global assessment. Lewis et al. have validated a non-invasive 9-point partial Mayo score (excluding endoscopy) and a 6-point partial Mayo score (composed of SF and RB) in a 12-week RCT; they also performed the full Mayo score (sensitivity and specificity over 80%) to identify the patient perceived clinical response [11]. Sanborne et al. have proposed and used a modified Mayo score (which excludes the subjectivity of the physical global assessment) in OCTAVE (induction 1 and 2; sustain) studies; it was consistent with the previously reported data using the original Mayo Score [12]. One of the outcome endpoints in LUCENT-1 and LUCENT-2 was symptomatic remission defined by SF = 0 or SF = 1 with ≥1-point decreased in modified Mayo score from baseline; RB = 0 [13].

Three main domains and preliminary set of criteria were proposed by Peyrin-Biroulet et al. relevant to the evaluation and classification of disease severity in IBD: impact of the disease on the patient (clinical symptoms, quality of life, fatigue, and disability), measurable disease burden (CRP, mucosal lesions, upper gastrointestinal involvement, and disease extent), and disease course (including structural damage, history/extension of intestinal resection, perianal disease, number of flares, and extraintestinal manifestations) [14].

With advanced therapeutics available for UC treatment, treatment targets beyond endoscopic improvement have emerged such as improvement of bowel urgency (BU). BU, the sudden need to have a bowel movement, is a frequent and bothersome core symptom of UC, experienced by up to 80% of patients, even in the absence of objective markers of active inflammation [15, 16]. BU is associated with a negative impact on patient's QoL [17]. Many UC patients consider controlling BU more important than SF or RB. Historically, BU was not used as an endpoint in clinical trials; if included it was reported only as binary (yes vs. no). *The Urgency* Numeric Rating Scale (NRS) was evaluated and validated in multicenter RCT with study sample of 1162 participants with moderate to severe UC; it is considered well-defined, content-valid, and reliable measurement of BU in adults with UC [18]. It can even document patient interpretation with modified recall periods (with 7-day or 3-day recall period) [19]. In LUCENT-1 and LUCENT-2 phase 3 studies, BU clinical meaningful improvement (≥3-point improvement from baseline) or BU remission (achieving a post-baseline score of 0 or 1) assessed by an 11-point urgency NRS (0 no urgency to 10 worst possible urgency) was associated with an improvement in QoL outcomes and PRO measures at week 12 which were sustained through week 52 [20].

2.2 Initiatives/guidelines

An initiative by the International Organization for the Study of IBD called STRIDE (Selecting Therapeutic Targets in Inflammatory Bowel Disease) in its 2021 update (STRIDE-II) added (using Delphi-like process and systematic literature review) clinical response (decrease of at least 50% in SF and RB) and then clinical remission (SF = 0 and RB = 0; or partial Mayo Score < 3 and no score > 1) with CRP normalization as minimal obligatory short-term (immediate) to medium-term (intermediate) treatment target [2]. Normalization of FC (to 100–250 mcg/g) was defined as another formal medium-term treatment target. Clinical remission in addition with objective improvement in non-invasive measures on inflammation must be shown.

ECCO-ESGAR guideline for diagnostic assessment in IBD defines the ideal monitoring test as non-invasive, simple to conduct, and easily interpretable [3]. CRP, FC, and IUS all have moderate to good responsiveness to changes in condition and high practicality, widely are available and well tolerated. Therefore, they could detect an imminent disease flare (often undetectable by symptom-based monitoring alone) and make provision for proactive treatment optimization.

AGA clinical practice guideline on the role of biomarkers for the management of UC suggests the use of non-invasive biomarkers (serum CRP, FC, and fecal lactoferrin [FL]) as an accurate, cheaper, and convenient first-line strategy (in combination with symptom-based monitoring) for monitoring UC patients in clinical remission as well as those with current symptoms [8]. For example, in asymptomatic patients without objective signs of active inflammation (FC <150 μg/g, normal FL, and/or normal CRP), routine endoscopic assessment of disease can be avoided. In patients with UC with moderate to severe symptoms, and objective signs of active ongoing inflammation (FC >150 μg/g, elevated FL, or elevated CRP), routine endoscopic assessment of disease to inform treatment decisions can also be avoided.

2.3 Serum markers

Currently, available serologic markers can be categorized into two primary groups: blood inflammatory biomarkers and IBD-related antibodies, some of which have prognostic, diagnostic, or even potential therapeutic significance.

2.3.1 C-reactive protein (CRP) and erythrocyte sedimentation rate (ESR)

Before the introduction of CRP into everyday clinical practice, ESR and thrombocytosis were used as a main inflammatory parameter. Notably, nowadays still in use, the Truelove and Witts Severity Index for UC includes ESR as one of its parameters [9].

CRP is an acute-phase reactant protein synthesized by the liver in response to interleukin-6 (IL-6) [21]. Although it has low specificity (many other conditions can cause increase such as infective gastroenteritis, ischemic colitis, appendicitis etc.), it is widely accepted as a reliable marker of inflammation in UC. Its short half-life of 16–24 hours makes it particularly responsive to changes in disease activity. Although CRP levels at diagnosis are related to the extent of the disease, a certain proportion of patients with mild forms of the disease have normal CRP levels [22, 23]. A CRP level of ≥12 mg/L predicts severe UC with 95% sensitivity and an 85% positive predictive value when used in place of ESR in the Truelove and Witts Severity Index for UC [23].

According to the literature, CRP levels tend to be higher in Crohn's disease (CD) compared to UC [24, 25]. However, the absolute concentration of CRP is not useful for differentiating between IBD types [22]. Anti-inflammatory or immunosuppressive drugs do not affect CRP production directly. Therefore, changes in CRP concentrations during treatment reflect the drug's effect on the underlying inflammation. Despite this, neither CRP nor ESR can be used as predictors of relapse in quiescent UC [26]. Conversely, CRP levels after the induction of biologic therapy may predict the long-term response to treatment [27, 28].

ESR is cheap and widely available test that measures the distance erythrocytes fall in 1 hour in a vertical column of non-coagulated blood under the influence of gravity [29]. Compared to CRP, ESR peaks more slowly, declines at a slower rate, and exhibits smaller changes in magnitude [22]. Compared to CRP, it has a slightly lower sensitivity [22] and lower correlation with endoscopic findings [30], but it remains a valuable parameter for disease diagnosis and monitoring.

2.3.2 Oncostatin M (OSM)

Oncostatin M (OSM), a cytokine within the interleukin-6 (IL-6) family, has attracted considerable attention for its role in UC, particularly regarding its impact on disease severity and treatment response.

OSM is produced in inflamed intestinal tissues and is linked to the pathogenesis of IBD. Its OSM receptor-β (OSMR) is expressed in nonhematopoietic, nonepithelial intestinal stromal cells, which respond to OSM by producing various proinflammatory molecules [31]. Elevated OSM levels have been observed in patients with active disease and correlate with histopathological severity and inflammation markers such as CRP and FC [31, 32]. Moreover, high levels of OSM before treatment are indicative of a poor response to anti-tumor necrosis factor (anti-TNF) therapies. According to Guo et al., patients with UC who have elevated OSM levels prior to treatment are less likely to achieve clinical remission after 1 year of therapy [33]. In a cross-sectional study by Verstockt et al., increased tissue and serum OSM were detected in newly diagnosed IBD patients and unaffected first-degree relatives of patients with IBD, while elevated colonic OSM and OSMR were associated with refractory disease phenotype such as requirement of biologic therapy within 2 years after diagnosis and primary nonresponse to both anti-TNF and vedolizumab therapy [34].

Due to its role in promoting intestinal inflammation and its link to treatment resistance, OSM is being investigated as a potential therapeutic target [31, 32].

2.3.3 Anti-Saccharomyces cerevisiae antibodies (ASCA) and perinuclear anti-neutrophil cytoplasmic antibodies (pANCA)

ASCAs are antibodies targeting the mannan heteropolymer found in the cell wall of *Saccharomyces cerevisiae*. Various studies have confirmed that ASCA has low sensitivity but high specificity for CD [35, 36]. It can be detected in patients with CD in up to 60–70% and in only 4% of patients with UC [37].

pANCA are autoantibodies targeting perinuclear cytoplasmic antigens in neutrophils. pANCA are primarily associated with rheumatological conditions and vasculitis. In the context of IBD, ANCA positivity ranges from 2% to 28% in patients with CD and 20–85% in patients with UC [36, 38].

In cases of indeterminate colitis, using a combination of antibodies can be more effective for establishing a definitive diagnosis. Bossiut et al. demonstrated that the combination of ASCA and p-ANCA is particularly useful in distinguishing CD from UC due to their distinct antibody patterns. Specifically, patients with CD are generally positive for ASCA and negative for p-ANCA, whereas patients with UC are positive for p-ANCA and negative for ASCA [39]. Neither pANCA nor ASCA are effective for monitoring disease activity. However, the presence of atypical p-ANCA has been associated with resistance to treatment in left-sided UC and an increased likelihood of early surgical intervention. Additionally, UC patients who are p-ANCA-positive and ASCA-negative at the initial infliximab infusion tend to experience a suboptimal early clinical response [22].

2.3.4 Anti-chitobioside carbohydrate IgA antibodies (ACCA), antilaminarbioside carbohydrate IgG antibodies (ALCA), and anti mannobioside carbohydrate IgG antibodies (AMCA)

Recent studies have focused on more anti-glycan antibodies in IBD, with ACCAs, ALCAs, and AMCAs emerging as effective diagnostic biomarkers for these conditions. Dotan et al. demonstrated that these biomarkers can effectively differentiate CD from UC with a specificity exceeding 90% [40].

Although the exact predictive value of ACCAs, ALCAs, and AMCAs specifically for treatment response in UC is still being studied, their presence could indicate variations in disease behavior and may influence treatment strategies. The combination of these antibodies with traditional markers (like pANCA and ASCA) could enhance diagnostic accuracy and help tailor therapeutic approaches for individual patients.

2.4 Fecal markers

Fecal biomarkers offer simple, non-invasive, and specific testing with possibilities of self-testing methods at home what is ideal for reducing number of unnecessary hospital visits [41]. Recently implemented T2T approach highlighted importance of biomarkers and their value in treatment optimization or treatment changes [42]. Several fecal biomarkers are discussed in detail in the following section.

2.4.1 Fecal calprotectin (FC)

FC is a calcium and zinc-binding protein found in neutrophils, monocytes, and macrophages. Its presence in feces is a marker of neutrophil-driven inflammation, making it particularly useful as a screening tool in detecting gastrointestinal inflammation [43]. FC is the most studied fecal biomarker, first quantified in 1992 [44]. Measuring FC levels is a non-invasive, cost-effective way to screen for and monitor intestinal inflammation, compared to more invasive procedures like endoscopy [41, 45]. FC is a stable protein that can persist in stool sample on room temperature for a week [45]. FC <50 μg/g (100 μg/g in children) is identified as a cut-off value which could exclude organic inflammation from irritable bowel syndrome (IBS). Significantly elevated FC levels (>250 μg/g) are detected in IBD. Moderately elevated FC (100–250 μg/g) can occur in some other GI conditions such as IBS, colorectal cancer (CRC), polyps, and celiac disease [46]. It is important to emphasize that elevated levels should be interpreted in the context of clinical signs, symptoms, and other diagnostic tests. It is generally used in the diagnosis and management of listed GI conditions:

IBD: Elevated FC levels are a strong indicator of intestinal inflammation associated with CD and UC. It also serves as a prognostic marker in IBD. Elevated levels are associated with active disease and can predict relapse in patients in remission (clinical and endoscopic) [41, 47]. Regular FC monitoring enables the detection of subclinical inflammation and early intervention before clinical symptoms worsen [48]. FC helps distinguish between IBD and IBS where normal levels of FC are expected [49]. For all those reasons, FC is included as a recommended monitoring fecal biomarker in clinical practice guidelines for UC.

CRC: FC has been recognized as a potential biomarker in the context of CRC since early 1990s [50]. There is a strong correlation between advanced CRC tumor stage, proximal tumor location and tumor type (mucinous), and elevated FC levels. Since high FC levels are indicative of inflammation and can be high in many other conditions, low specificity prevents it for being used for CRC screening [51, 52].

2.4.2 Fecal lactoferrin (FL)

FL is another investigated fecal biomarker of intestinal inflammation. It is an iron-binding glycoprotein present in feces. Its main function is transporting iron Fe^{3+} to blood stream. FL has bactericidal role since it limits iron availability. It influences deregulated gut microbiota composition in IBD patients by eliminating harmful bacteria and promoting beneficial bacterial growth [53]. FL is released by activated neutrophils and phagocytic cells during inflammation [41]. Like FC, FL levels are elevated in IBD. High LF levels suggest further evaluation for either IBD or infectious diseases, while normal levels indicate that symptoms are more likely functional. FL can help predict IBD recurrence and guide treatment adjustments [54]. It can be easily tested from liquid or solid samples with immunoassay tests. FL is stabile in room temperature samples even longer than then FC (2 weeks). Commercial tests simplify the use of LF as a biomarker and reduce the number of hospital visits. One precisely defined cut-off value (7.25 μg/g) which is identical for all laboratories is an advantage of FL testing [55].

An elevated FL level has been reported in the population of patients with CRC in comparison with healthy controls, but FL cannot be recommended as a CRC diagnostic tool. Persistent elevation of FL in IBD patients may indicate the development of dysplasia or carcinoma and should be promptly evaluated [53].

2.4.3 Lipocalin 2

Lipocalin 2 (LCN2), also known as neutrophil gelatinase-associated lipocalin (NGAL), or siderocalin, is a protein involved in immune responses, discovered in 1989. It has been recently shown to play a role in regulating intestinal inflammation. It is released by macrophages and neutrophils during inflammation, but also from colonic epithelial cells which made him interesting as a potential biomarker [56, 57]. Research indicate LCN2 has influence on gut microbiota and modulates the inflammation, potentially contributing to the pathogenesis of IBD. It serves as a significant biomarker especially for patients with active UC [56]. LCN2 correlates with clinical and endoscopic disease activity. It has shown comparable sensitivity and specificity to fecal FC [57]. While both UC and CRC can elevate lipocalin 2 levels, the degree and pattern of elevation can differ. UC typically causes a more consistent and significant rise in lipocalin 2 due to chronic inflammation. Expression level of LCN2 was significantly negatively correlated with UC disease duration and UC-associated carcinogenesis in a study by Kou et al. [58]. Diagnostic performances of biomarkers are summarized in **Table 1**.

2.5 Imaging methods

2.5.1 Intestinal ultrasound (IUS) and other imaging methods in diagnosis and management of ulcerative colitis

Standard imaging methods are usually second-line procedures in the context of UC. Plain radiography and abdominal CT are usually performed in the emergency

	Specificity	Sensitivity	PPV	NPV
CRP cut-off 1.2–7.3 mg/L for active disease [8]	77%	63%		
CRP cut-off 12 mg/L for ASUC [23]	90.3%	95%	85%	92.8%
Fecal calprotectin cut-off 150 ± 50 mcg/g [8]	69%	71%		
Fecal lactoferin cut-off 7.25 mcg/g [8]	75%	83%		
Oncostatin M cut-off 118.50 pg/mL for active disease [59]	54.2%	66.7%		
pANCA for establishment of diagnose [60]	94.3%	53.7%	81.5%	81.4%
CD vs. UC [60]				
ASCA+	58.5%	66.2%	73.4%	50%
ASCA+/pANCA–	80.5%	50.7%	81.8%	51.5%
UC vs. CD [60]				
pANCA+	78.9%	53.7%	59.5%	74.7%
pANCA+/ASCA–	94.4%	31.7%	76.5%	70.5%
ALCA in differentiating CD vs. UC [61]	92.3%	25.6%	90.3%	30.8%
AMCA in differentiating CD vs. UC [61]	93.1%	27.3%	91.7%	31.4%
ACCA in differentiating CD vs. UC [61]	93.1%	16.8%	87.1%	28.6%

Table 1.
Diagnostic performances of UC biomarkers.

setting to rule perforation or toxic megacolon but are of limited use in long-term monitoring due to radiation exposure. MR enterography (MRE), although shown to be accurate in assessing and monitoring UC, is rarely used in clinical practice due to its long duration, expensiveness, reduced availability, and poor tolerability, as bowel preparation and intravenous contrast agents are needed [62]. MRE is mostly used to detect signs of small bowel involvement in indeterminate IBD.

IUS is an emerging method in the evaluation of the bowel. Recognizing the invasive nature of endoscopy as the gold standard of UC diagnosis and monitoring, non-invasive methods such as IUS show promise in reducing the need for invasive procedures. Through the advancements in technology and increasing availability of ultrasound machines this method is pushing into the frontlines of care for IBD patients.

Bowel wall thickness (BWT) greater than 3 mm as measure with intestinal ultrasound is considered significant and can indicate an inflammatory process. A linear mid-to-high frequency ultrasound probe is used to evaluate the entire length of the bowel in greater detail, while a convex low-to-mid frequency probe is usually used to evaluate deeper seated bowel loops and the rectum. The color doppler signal (CDS) in the bowel wall can be graded semi-quantitatively from non-existent to a spot like pattern, long stretches in the bowel wall, and long stretches extending into the mesentery.

The fundamentals of an IUS examinations in the form of recommendations and guidelines have been published by the European Federation of Societies for Ultrasound in Medicine and Biology in 2018 [63].

Key topics to address on the role of IUS in UC are the ability to diagnose the disease, evaluation and scoring of severity and extent, monitoring treatment response, and detecting complications. Special scenarios such as pregnancy and severe acute colitis are also discussed.

2.5.2 The role of IUS in diagnosing UC

The diagnosis of UC relies on endoscopy and clinical characteristics of the disease and cannot be based solely on imaging findings. The hallmarks of UC on IUS are BWT and the presence of CDS. The loss of bowel wall stratification as well as the presence of inflammatory fat can indicate the severity of the inflammation.

A systemic review and meta-analysis determined the accuracy for evaluation of individual colorectal segments in patients with IBD. The results showed that bowel wall thickness ≥3 mm identified inflamed colonic segments with 86.4% pooled sensitivity and 88.3% specificity. When used for the rectum, the same cut-off yielded 74.5% sensitivity and 69.5% specificity [64].

2.5.3 Monitoring UC using IUS

The TRUST&UC study was among the first to establish IUS as a monitoring tool in UC. The study showed significant decrease of BWT in response to therapy starting at the 2-week timepoint. Normalization of the BWT at 12 weeks (sigmoid colon 32.0%; descending colon 37.6%) highly correlated with clinical response [65]. Further studies have shown that IUS parameters at week 6 of initiating therapy predicted endoscopic remission at 26 weeks [66].

2.5.4 IUS scoring systems in UC

Several scoring systems have been developed for IUS use in UC. One of the most used is the Milan ultrasound criteria (MUC), computed according to the following mathematical formula: 1.4 × BWT (mm) + 2 × bowel wall flow (1 if present or 0 if absent). The MUC > 6.2 discriminates active vs. inactive UC and has been validated in independent studies [67].

2.5.5 IUS in special situations in patients with UC

2.5.5.1 Pregnancy

IUS is of special value in pregnancy where most of the colon can be visualized during the first and second trimester. It helps with the diagnosis as well as visualizing the extent of inflammation and can be used as a monitoring tool. The feasibility of IUS decreases in the third trimester due to the limited visualization of the sigmoid colon. It remains however a reproducible non-invasive method of obtaining information on the activity and extent of the disease as well as response to treatment during pregnancy [68].

2.5.5.2 Severe acute UC

A severe flare-up of UC can be a life-threatening condition that is typically treated with high-dose corticosteroids and/or anti-TNF. A recent study showed that BWT measured 48 hours after intravenous corticosteroid initiation predicted risk of colectomy. IUS can be used to early identify steroid non-responders and accelerate escalation of therapy [69].

2.6 Time frames for clinical, biochemical, and imaging assessments

The optimal non-invasive, patient-centered monitoring time interval for follow up of UC patients is still under debate. In symptomatic UC patient with active disease repeat clinical and biochemical (CRP, FC, and FL) assessment to determine response to treatment can be reasonable alternative to endoscopy and should be performed 3–6 months after treatment initiation/adjustment (according to ECCO-ESGAR, STRIDE-II, and AGA) [2, 3, 8]. In clinically asymptomatic patients with elevated serum and/or stool markers of inflammation, AGA suggests endoscopic assessment of disease activity, although repeat measurement of biomarkers in 3–6 months interval can be a reasonable alternative. Also, in UC patients with mild symptoms (slight increase in SF and/or infrequent RB) and normal biomarkers of inflammation repeat measurement of biomarkers in 3–6 months may be a reasonable alternative in patients who prefer to avoid endoscopic assessment or empiric treatment escalation. In UC patients who have reached clinical and biochemical remission depending upon duration of remission and current therapy, ECCO-ESGAR recommends clinical and biochemical assessment in 3–6 months; on the other hand, in the group of UC patients with symptomatic remission, AGA suggests monitoring strategy that combines symptoms and biomarkers with interval biomarker monitoring that should be performed every 6–12 months.

The use of IUS in combination with biomarkers to monitor disease activity seems like a reasonable postulate. Point-of-care IUS offers an additional benefit for rapid, early, replicable, and non-invasive assessment of a subset of patients with highly active/difficult-to-treat/steroid refractory UC [69]. The International Bowel Ultrasound Group suggests that, after baseline IUS, response to treatment initiation/escalation/change should be evaluated with IUS at week 14 ± 2, and between weeks 26 and 52, or IUS should be repeated depending on clinical and/or biochemical suspicion of UC flare [70]. Kucharzik et al. even suggest early combined (PROs and repeated IUS) assessment of treatment response 2–4 weeks after treatment initiation/escalation/change depending on UC activity followed by monitoring strategy that combines PROs, FC, and IUS at month 3; PROs, FC, IUS and endoscopy at month 6; and PROs, FC and IUS at month 12 [71]. The proposed timetable for UC assessment in clinical practice is shown in **Figure 1**.

2.7 Cost-effectiveness of non-invasive monitoring

Cortesi et al. have assessed the cost-effectiveness of a T2T approach based on the normalization of clinical signs and FC using a decision analytical Markov model which included five treatment lines and was conducted from the Italian National Health Service perspective using a 3-year time horizon [72]. Combination of symptom- and biomarker-based T2T approach resulted in an increased time spent by a mild-moderate UC patients in clinical remission and reduced incidence of UC relapse but was associated with higher costs.

2.8 Open questions

BU should be considered as a third PRO in UC along with SF and RB and should be included as a T2T treatment target in future guidelines.

Regulatory agencies have embraced recent shift toward evaluating PROs (as a co-primary endpoint in clinical drug trials) because patients' perceptions of their illness and symptoms may differ significantly from those of the treating physician [73]. But

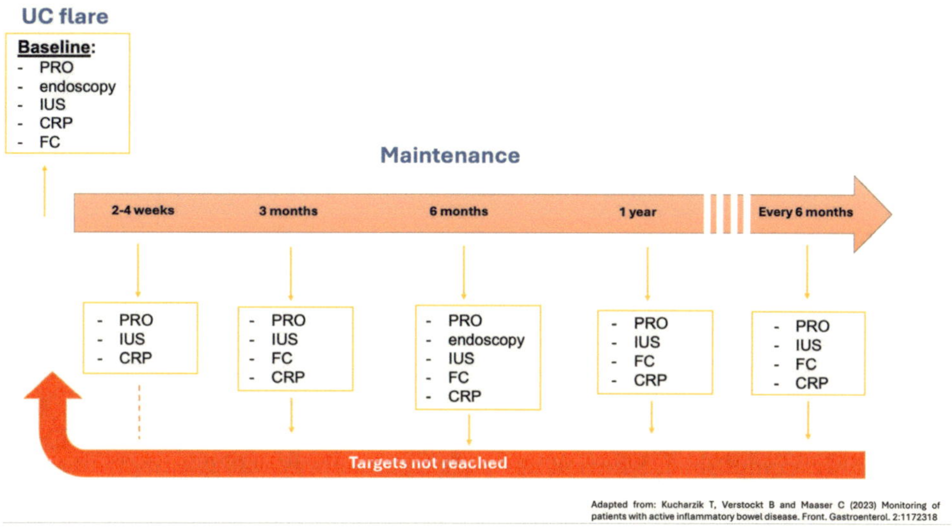

Figure 1.
Potential timetable for UC assessment in clinical practice.

we all should be aware that PROs and clinical activity systems derived from them are highly subjective with dubious correlation with inflammation and can be potentially influenced by other causes (diet, anatomy, IBS, ADD, and microbiome).

When comparing diagnostic performance of biomarkers with endoscopy, we should know that FC has high sensitivity and lower specificity in identifying mucosal inflammation, and CRP has the opposite characteristics: it has higher specificity but low sensitivity [74].

There is inter-individual heterogeneity in biomarker responsiveness. In population with SNP polymorphisms in the CRP gene (prevalence of the non-wild type of status is 10–15% in general population with an additional 30–35% having heterozygosity at these loci), lower degree of CRP elevation is expected, and the performance of CRP as a biomarker may be less reliable [75, 76].

Fecal biomarkers assays may not be interchangeable (inter- and intra-assay test variability); the same assay should be used for a particular patient in longitudinal observation.

There is still an open question about the accuracy of different FC cutoffs for ruling out the endoscopically active disease. The guideline panel behind AGA guidelines chose a FC cut-off (<150 μg/g) that is broadly applicable across a wide range of UC clinical scenarios, rather than reporting multiple different cut-offs for different scenarios [8].

There are limited studies on different cut-offs for LF; for now, positive (elevated) or negative LF, corresponding to a cut-off of 7.25 μg/g is advocated [8].

It is advised to compare the serum and/or fecal biomarkers at the time of endoscopic evaluation to determine their correlation in an individual patient.

In a study by Barsky et al., 60% of IBD patients initially preferred fecal markers over endoscopy; most study participants changed their choice to colonoscopy after learning more about the accuracy of currently available fecal markers for disease monitoring [77].

FC's high cost, absence of widespread availability, and low patient adherence still limits its use as a potential surrogate for endoscopy.

Although there are some interesting data, biomarkers and IUS cannot replace endoscopy for detection and surveillance of UC-associated carcinogenesis.

One of the most important knowledge gaps that needs to be addressed in translating guidelines to clinical practice is the lack of specific biomarkers to aid with predicting individual patient response to specific therapies.

3. Conclusions

Non-invasive strategy for management of UC, that combines interval symptom- and (serum and fecal) biomarker-based monitoring with new diagnostic modalities such as IUS, is now recognized and established in new diagnostic algorithms that guide treatment decisions. By placing emphasis on fast patient-centered evaluation, a reduction in the number of unnecessary invasive procedures such as endoscopy can be easily accomplished. Relevant up-to-date guidance is available to practicing IBD specialists; it is time to translate its full potential to real life. Cost-effectiveness studies demonstrating which non-invasive diagnostic modality/monitoring strategy is best are required. Further clinical trials and real-world clinical studies are needed to convince insurers that covering non-invasive-based monitoring will improve patient satisfaction and clinical outcomes.

Conflict of interest

The authors declare no conflict of interest.

Author details

Vedran Tomašić[1]*, Alen Biščanin[1,2], Dominik Kralj[3], Petra Ćaćić[3] and Doris Ogresta[3]

1 Department of Endoscopy and Day Hospital, Sestre Milosrdnice University Hospital Centre, Zagreb, Croatia

2 University of Zagreb School of Medicine, Zagreb, Croatia

3 Department of Gastroenterology and Hepatology, Sestre Milosrdnice University Hospital Centre, Zagreb, Croatia

*Address all correspondence to: tomasicvedran@gmail.com

References

[1] Kobayashi T, Siegmund B, Le Berre C, Wei SC, Ferrante M, Shen B, et al. Ulcerative colitis. Nature Reviews. Disease Primers. 2020;**6**(1):74. DOI: 10.1038/s41572-020-0205-x

[2] Turner D, Ricciuto A, Lewis A, D'Amico F, Dhaliwal J, Griffiths AM, et al. STRIDE-II: An update on the selecting therapeutic targets in inflammatory bowel disease (STRIDE) initiative of the International Organization for the Study of IBD (IOIBD): Determining therapeutic goals for treat-to-target strategies in IBD. Gastroenterology. 2021;**160**(5):1570-1583. DOI: 10.1053/j.gastro.2020.12.031. Epub 2021 Feb 19

[3] Maaser C, Sturm A, Vavricka SR, Kucharzik T, Fiorino G, Annese V, et al. ECCO-ESGAR guideline for diagnostic assessment in IBD part 1: Initial diagnosis, monitoring of known IBD, detection of complications. Journal of Crohn's & Colitis. 2019;**13**(2):144-164. DOI: 10.1093/ecco-jcc/jjy113

[4] Raine T, Bonovas S, Burisch J, Kucharzik T, Adamina M, Annese V, et al. ECCO guidelines on therapeutics in ulcerative colitis: Medical treatment. Journal of Crohn's & Colitis. 2022;**16**(1):2-17. DOI: 10.1093/ecco-jcc/jjab178

[5] Okobi OE, Udoete IO, Fasehun OO, Okobi T, Evbayekha EO, Ekabua JJ, et al. A review of four practice guidelines of inflammatory bowel disease. Cureus. 2021;**13**(8):e16859. DOI: 10.7759/cureus.16859

[6] Buie MJ, Coward S, Shaheen AA, Holroyd-Leduc J, Hracs L, Ma C, et al. Hospitalization rates for inflammatory bowel disease are decreasing over time: A population-based cohort study. Inflammatory Bowel Diseases. 2023;**29**(10):1536-1545. DOI: 10.1093/ibd/izad020

[7] Goodsall TM, Noy R, Nguyen TM, Costello SP, Jairath V, Bryant RV. Systematic review: Patient perceptions of monitoring tools in inflammatory bowel disease. Journal of the Canadian Association of Gastroenterology. 2020;**4**(2):e31-e41. DOI: 10.1093/jcag/gwaa001

[8] Singh S, Ananthakrishnan AN, Nguyen NH, Cohen BL, Velayos FS, Weiss JM, et al. AGA clinical practice guideline on the role of biomarkers for the management of ulcerative colitis. Gastroenterology. 2023;**164**(3):344-372. DOI: 10.1053/j.gastro.2022.12.007

[9] Truelove SC, Witts LJ. Cortisone in ulcerative colitis; final report on a therapeutic trial. British Medical Journal. 1955;**2**(4947):1041-1048. DOI: 10.1136/bmj.2.4947.1041

[10] Schroeder KW, Tremaine WJ, Ilstrup DM. Coated oral 5-aminosalicylic acid therapy for mildly to moderately active ulcerative colitis. A randomized study. The New England Journal of Medicine. 1987;**317**(26):1625-1629. DOI: 10.1056/NEJM198712243172603

[11] Lewis JD, Chuai S, Nessel L, Lichtenstein GR, Aberra FN, Ellenberg JH. Use of the noninvasive components of the Mayo score to assess clinical response in ulcerative colitis. Inflammatory Bowel Diseases. 2008;**14**(12):1660-1666. DOI: 10.1002/ibd.20520

[12] Sandborn WJ, Sands BE, Vermeire S, Leung Y, Guo X, Modesto I, et al.

Modified Mayo score versus Mayo score for evaluation of treatment efficacy in patients with ulcerative colitis: Data from the tofacitinib OCTAVE program. Therapeutic Advances in Gastroenterology. 2022;**15**:17562848221136331. DOI: 10.1177/17562848221136331

[13] Sands BE, D'Haens G, Clemow DB, Irwing PM, Johns JT, Hunter Gibble T, et al. Two-year efficacy and safety of Mirikizumab following 104 weeks of continuous treatment: Interim results from the LUCENT-3 open-label extension study (ulcerative colitis). Gastroenterology and Hepatology (New York). 2023;**19**(12 Suppl 9):10-11

[14] Peyrin-Biroulet L, Panés J, Sandborn WJ, Vermeire S, Danese S, Feagan BG, et al. Defining disease severity in inflammatory bowel diseases: Current and future directions. Clinical Gastroenterology and Hepatology. 2016;**14**(3):348-354.e17. DOI: 10.1016/j.cgh.2015.06.001 Epub 2015

[15] Newton L, Randall JA, Hunter T, Keith S, Symonds T, Secrest RJ, et al. A qualitative study exploring the health-related quality of life and symptomatic experiences of adults and adolescents with ulcerative colitis. Journal of Patient-Reported Outcomes. 2019;**3**(1):66. DOI: 10.1186/s41687-019-0154-x

[16] Dawwas GK, Jajeh H, Shan M, Naegeli AN, Hunter T, Lewis JD. Prevalence and factors associated with fecal urgency among patients with ulcerative colitis and Crohn's disease in the study of a prospective adult research cohort with inflammatory bowel disease. Crohn's & Colitis 360. 2021;**3**(3):otab046. DOI: 10.1093/crocol/otab046

[17] Long MD, Schreiber S, Hibi T, Gibble TH, Fisher DA, Park G, et al. Association of bowel urgency with quality-of-life measures in patients with moderately-to-severely active ulcerative colitis: Results from phase 3 LUCENT-1 (induction) and LUCENT-2 (maintenance) studies. Crohn's & Colitis 360. 2024;**6**(1):otae001. DOI: 10.1093/crocol/otae001

[18] Dubinsky MC, Shan M, Delbecque L, Lissoos T, Hunter T, Harding G, et al. Psychometric evaluation of the urgency NRS as a new patient-reported outcome measure for patients with ulcerative colitis. Journal of Patient-Reported Outcomes. 2022;**6**(1):114. DOI: 10.1186/s41687-022-00522-2

[19] Jairath V, Gibble TH, Moses R, Klooster B, Litcher-Kelly L, Walker M, et al. Patient interpretations of patient-reported outcome measures to assess bowel urgency: Qualitative interviews in ulcerative colitis. Journal of Patient-Reported Outcomes. 2024;**8**(1):54. DOI: 10.1186/s41687-024-00733-9

[20] Sands BE, Feagan BG, Hunter Gibble T, Traxler KA, Morris N, Eastman WJ, et al. Mirikizumab improves quality of life in patients with moderately-to-severely active ulcerative colitis: Results from the phase 3 LUCENT-1 induction and LUCENT-2 maintenance studies. Crohn's & Colitis 360. 2023;**5**(4):otad070. DOI: 10.1093/crocol/otad070

[21] Nehring SM, Goyal A, Patel BC. C Reactive Protein. Treasure Island (FL): StatPearls Publishing; 2023. Available from: http://europepmc.org/books/NBK441843

[22] Cioffi M, De RA, Serao R, Picone I, Vietri MT. Laboratory markers in ulcerative colitis: Current insights and future advances. World Journal of Gastrointestinal Pathophysiology. 2015;**6**(1):13-22

[23] Croft A, Lord A, Radford-Smith G. Markers of systemic inflammation in acute attacks of ulcerative colitis: What level of C-reactive protein constitutes severe colitis? Journal of Crohn's & Colitis. 2022;**16**(7):1089-1096

[24] Gross V, Andus T, Caesar I, Roth M, Schölmerich J. Evidence for continuous stimulation of interleukin-6 production in Crohn's disease. Gastroenterology. 1992;**102**(2):514-519

[25] Niederau C, Backmerhoff F, Schumacher B, Niederau C. Inflammatory mediators and acute phase proteins in patients with Crohn's disease and ulcerative colitis. Hepato-Gastroenterology. 1997;**44**(13):90-107

[26] Bitton A, Peppercorn MA, Antonioli DA, Niles JL, Shah S, Bousvaros A, et al. Clinical, biological, and histologic parameters as predictors of relapse in ulcerative colitis. Gastroenterology. 2001;**120**(1):13-20

[27] Iwasa R, Yamada A, Sono K, Furukawa R, Takeuchi K, Suzuki Y. C-reactive protein level at 2 weeks following initiation of infliximab induction therapy predicts outcomes in patients with ulcerative colitis: A 3 year follow-up study. BMC Gastroenterology. 2015;**15**:103

[28] Cornillie F, Hanauer SB, Diamond RH, Wang J, Tang KL, Xu Z, et al. Postinduction serum infliximab trough level and decrease of C-reactive protein level are associated with durable sustained response to infliximab: A retrospective analysis of the ACCENT I trial. Gut. 2014;**63**(11):1721-1727

[29] Gabay C, Kushner I. Acute-phase proteins and other systemic responses to inflammation. The New England Journal of Medicine. 1999;**340**(6):448-454

[30] Turner D, Mack DR, Hyams J, LeLeiko N, Otley A, Markowitz J, et al. C-reactive protein (CRP), erythrocyte sedimentation rate (ESR) or both? A systematic evaluation in pediatric ulcerative colitis. Journal of Crohn's & Colitis. 2011;**5**(5):423-429

[31] West NR, Hegazy AN, Owens BMJ, Bullers SJ, Linggi B, Buonocore S, et al. Oncostatin M drives intestinal inflammation and predicts response to tumor necrosis factor-neutralizing therapy in patients with inflammatory bowel disease. Nature Medicine. 2017;**23**(5):579-589

[32] Yang Y, Fu K-Z, Pan G. Role of Oncostatin M in the prognosis of inflammatory bowel disease: A meta-analysis. World Journal of Gastrointestinal Surgery. 2024;**16**(1):228-238

[33] Guo A, Ross C, Chande N, Gregor J, Ponich T, Khanna R, et al. High oncostatin M predicts lack of clinical remission for patients with inflammatory bowel disease on tumor necrosis factor α antagonists. Scientific Reports. 2022;**12**(1):1185

[34] Verstock S, Verstockt B, Machiels K, Vancamelbeke M, Ferrante M, Cleynen I, et al. Oncostatin M is biomarker of diagnosis, worse disease prognosis, and therapeutic nonresponse in inflammatory bowel disease. Inflammatory Bowel Disease. 2021;**27**(10):1564-1575

[35] Reese GE, Constantinides VA, Simillis C, Darzi AW, Orchard TR, Fazio VW, et al. Diagnostic precision of anti-*Saccharomyces cerevisiae* antibodies and perinuclear antineutrophil cytoplasmic antibodies in inflammatory bowel disease. The American Journal of Gastroenterology. 2006;**101**(10):2410-2422

[36] Joossens S, Reinisch W, Vermeire S, Sendid B, Poulain D, Peeters M, et al.

The value of serologic markers in indeterminate colitis: A prospective follow-up study. Gastroenterology. 2002;**122**(5):1242-1247

[37] Peyrin-Biroulet L, Standaert-Vitse A, Branche J, Chamaillard M. IBD serological panels: Facts and perspectives. Inflammatory Bowel Diseases. 2007;**13**(12):1561-1566

[38] Bossuyt X. Serologic markers in inflammatory bowel disease. Clinical Chemistry. 2006;**52**(2):171-181

[39] Dotan I. New serologic markers for inflammatory bowel disease diagnosis. Digestive Diseases. 2010;**28**(3):418-423

[40] Dotan I, Fishman S, Dgani Y, Schwartz M, Karban A, Lerner A, et al. Antibodies against laminaribioside and chitobioside are novel serologic markers in Crohn's disease. Gastroenterology. 2006;**131**(2):366-378

[41] Bencardino S, D'Amico F, Zilli A, Parigi TL, Alloca M, Fiorino G, et al. Fecal, blood, and urinary biomarkers in inflammatory bowel disease. Journal of Translational Gastroenterology. 2024;**2**(2):61-75. DOI: 10.14218/JTG.2024.00001

[42] Garcia NM, Cohen NA, Rubin DT. Treat-to-target and sequencing therapies in Crohn's disease. United European Gastroenterology Journal. 2022;**10**(10):1121-1128. DOI: 10.1002/ueg2.12336

[43] Ayling RM, Kok K. Fecal calprotectin. Advances in Clinical Chemistry. 2018;**87**:161-190. DOI: 10.1016/bs.acc.2018.07.005. Epub 2018

[44] Røseth AG, Fagerhol MK, Aadland E, Schjønsby H. Assessment of the neutrophil dominating protein calprotectin in feces. A methodologic study. Scandinavian Journal of Gastroenterology. 1992;**27**(9):793-798. DOI: 10.3109/00365529209011186

[45] Liu D, Saikam V, Skrada KA, Merlin D, Iyer SS. Inflammatory bowel disease biomarkers. Medicinal Research Reviews. 2022;**42**(5):1856-1887. DOI: 10.1002/med.21893. Epub 2022 May 23

[46] Bjarnason I. The use of fecal calprotectin in inflammatory bowel disease. Gastroenterology and Hepatology (New York). 2017;**13**(1):53-56

[47] Wagatsuma K, Yokoyama Y, Nakase H. Role of biomarkers in the diagnosis and treatment of inflammatory bowel disease. Life (Basel). 2021;**11**(12):1375. DOI: 10.3390/life11121375

[48] Kostas A, Siakavellas SI, Kosmidis C, Takou A, Nikou J, Maropoulos G, et al. Fecal calprotectin measurement is a marker of short-term clinical outcome and presence of mucosal healing in patients with inflammatory bowel disease. World Journal of Gastroenterology. 2017;**23**(41):7387-7396. DOI: 10.3748/wjg.v23.i41.7387

[49] Waugh N, Cummins E, Royle P, Kandala NB, Shyangdan D, Arasaradnam R, et al. Faecal calprotectin testing for differentiating amongst inflammatory and non-inflammatory bowel diseases: Systematic review and economic evaluation. Health Technology Assessment. 2013;**17**(55):xv-xix, 1-211. DOI: 10.3310/hta17550

[50] Roseth AG, Fagerhol MK, Aadland E, Schjonsby H. Assessment of the neutrophil dominating protein calprotectin in feces. A methodologic study. Scandinavian Journal of Gastroenterology. 1992;**27**(9):793-798.

DOI: 10.3109/00365529209011186.ID: PMC4781415

[51] Ross FA, Park JH, Mansouri D, Combet E, Horgan PG, McMillan DC, et al. The role of faecal calprotectin in diagnosis and staging of colorectal neoplasia: A systematic review and meta-analysis. BMC Gastroenterology. 2022;**22**(1):176. DOI: 10.1186/s12876-022-02220-1

[52] Blad N, Palmqvist R, Karling P. Pre-diagnostic faecal calprotectin levels in patients with colorectal cancer: A retrospective study. BMC Cancer. 2022;**22**(1):315. DOI: 10.1186/s12885-022-09440-4

[53] Cutone A, Ianiro G, Lepanto MS, Rosa L, Valenti P, Bonaccorsi di Patti MC, et al. Lactoferrin in the prevention and treatment of intestinal inflammatory pathologies associated with colorectal cancer development. Cancers (Basel). 2020;**12**(12):3806. DOI: 10.3390/cancers12123806

[54] Siddiqui I, Majid H, Abid S. Update on clinical and research application of fecal biomarkers for gastrointestinal diseases. World Journal of Gastrointestinal Pharmacology and Therapeutics. 2017;**8**(1):39-46. DOI: 10.4292/wjgpt.v8.i1.39

[55] Abraham BP. Fecal lactoferrin testing. Gastroenterology and Hepatology (New York). 2018;**14**(12):713-716

[56] Stallhofer J, Friedrich M, Konrad-Zerna A, Wetzke M, Lohse P, Glas J, et al. Lipocalin-2 is a disease activity marker in inflammatory bowel disease regulated by IL-17A, IL-22, and TNF-α and modulated by IL23R genotype status. Inflammatory Bowel Diseases. 2015;**21**(10):2327-2340. DOI: 10.1097/MIB.0000000000000515

[57] Zollner A, Schmiderer A, Reider SJ, Oberhuber G, Pfister A, Texler B, et al. Faecal biomarkers in inflammatory bowel diseases: Calprotectin versus lipocalin-2-a comparative study. Journal of Crohn's & Colitis. 2021;**15**(1):43-54. DOI: 10.1093/ecco-jcc/jjaa124

[58] Kou F, Cheng Y, Shi L, Liu J, Liu Y, Shi R, et al. LCN2 as a potential diagnostic biomarker for ulcerative colitis-associated carcinogenesis related to disease duration. Frontiers in Oncology. 2022;**11**:793760. DOI: 10.3389/fonc.2021.793760

[59] Mohamed GA, El-Latif Mohamed HA, Halima ASA, Elshaarawy MEA, Khedr A. Changes in serum Oncostatin M levels during treatment of inflammatory bowel disease; the Egyptian. Journal of Hospital Medicine. 2022;**89**(2):7217-7225

[60] Wang Z, Shi K, Peng J. Serologic testing of a panel of five antibodies in inflammatory bowel diseases: Diagnostic value and correlation with disease phenotype. Biomedical Reports. 2017;**6**:401-410. DOI: 10.3892/br.2017.860

[61] Rieder F, Schleder S, Wolf A, Dirmeier A, Strauch U, Obermeier F, et al. Association of the novel serologic anti-glycan antibodies anti-laminarin and anti-chitin with complicated Crohn's disease behavior. Inflammatory Bowel Diseases. 2010;**16**(2):263-274. DOI: 10.1002/ibd.21046

[62] Alfarone L, Dal Buono A, Craviotto V, Zilli A, Fiorino G, Furfaro F, et al. Cross-Sectional Imaging Instead of Colonoscopy in Inflammatory Bowel Diseases: Lights and Shadows. Journal of Clinical Medicine. 2022;**11**(2):353. DOI: 10.3390/jcm11020353

[63] Maconi G, Nylund K, Ripolles T, Calabrese E, Dirks K, Dietrich CF, et al. EFSUMB recommendations and clinical

guidelines for intestinal ultrasound (GIUS) in inflammatory bowel diseases. Ultraschall in der Medizin. 2018;**39**(3):304-317

[64] Sagami S, Kobayashi T, Miyatani Y, Okabayashi S, Yamazaki H, Takada T, et al. Accuracy of ultrasound for evaluation of colorectal segments in patients with inflammatory bowel diseases: A systematic review and meta-analysis. Clinical Gastroenterology and Hepatology. 2021;**19**(5):908-921.e6

[65] Maaser C, Petersen F, Helwig U, Fisher I, Roessler A, Rath S, et al. Intestinal ultrasound for monitoring therapeutic response in patients with ulcerative colitis: Results from the TRUST and UC study. Gut. 2020;**69**:1629-1636

[66] de Voogd FA, Bots SJ, van Wassenaer EA, de Jong M, Pruijt MJ, D'Haens GR, et al. Early intestinal ultrasound predicts clinical and endoscopic treatment response and demonstrates drug-specific kinetics in moderate-to-severe ulcerative colitis. Inflammatory Bowel Diseases. 2023:izad274. DOI: 10.1093/ibd/izad274. [Epub ahead of print]

[67] Allocca M, Filippi E, Costantino A, Bonovas S, Fiorino G, Furfaro F, et al. Milan ultrasound criteria are accurate in assessing disease activity in ulcerative colitis: External validation. United European Gastroenterology Journal. 2021;**9**(4):438-442

[68] de Voogd FA, Joshi H, Van Wassenaer E, Bots S, D'Haens G, Gecse K. Intestinal ultrasound to evaluate treatment response during pregnancy in patients with inflammatory bowel disease. Inflammatory Bowel Diseases. 2022;**28**(7):1045-1052. DOI: 10.1093/ibd/izab216

[69] Ilvemark JFKF, Wilkens R, Thielsen P, Dige A, Boysen T, Brynskov J, et al. Early intestinal ultrasound in severe ulcerative colitis identifies patients at increased risk of 1-year treatment failure and colectomy. Journal of Crohn's & Colitis. 2024;**2024**:jjae101. DOI: 10.1093/ecco-jcc/jjae101. Epub ahead of print

[70] Ilvemark JFKF, Hansen T, Goodsall TM, Seidelin JB, Al-Farhan H, Allocca M, et al. Defining transabdominal intestinal ultrasound treatment response and remission in inflammatory bowel disease: Systematic review and expert consensus statement. Journal of Crohn's & Colitis. 2022;**16**(4):554-580. DOI: 10.1093/ecco-jcc/jjab173

[71] Kucharzik T, Verstockt B, Maaser C. Monitoring of patients with active inflammatory bowel disease. Frontiers in Gastroenterology. 2023;**2**. DOI: 10.3389/fgstr.2023.1172318

[72] Cortesi PA, Fiorino G, Peyrin-Biroulet L, Mantovani LG, Jairath V, Paridaens K, et al. Non-invasive monitoring and treat-to-target approach are cost-effective in patients with mild-moderate ulcerative colitis. Alimentary Pharmacology & Therapeutics. 2023;**57**(5):486-495. DOI: 10.1111/apt.17261

[73] Rochelle TL, Fidler H. The importance of illness perceptions, quality of life and psychological status in patients with ulcerative colitis and Crohn's disease. Journal of Health Psychology. 2013;**18**:972-983

[74] Mosli MH, Zou G, Garg SK, Feagan SG, MacDonald JK, Chande N, et al. C-reactive protein, fecal calprotectin, and stool lactoferrin for detection of endoscopic activity in symptomatic inflammatory bowel disease patients: A systematic review and meta-analysis. The American Journal of Gastroenterology. 2015;**110**:802-819; quiz 820

[75] Henderson P, Kennedy NA, Van Limbergen JE, Cameron FL, Satsangi J, Russell RK, et al. Serum C-reactive protein and CRP genotype in pediatric inflammatory bowel disease: Influence on phenotype, natural history, and response to therapy. Inflammatory Bowel Diseases. 2015;**21**:596-605

[76] Moran CJ, Kaplan JL, Winter HS. Genetic variation affects C-reactive protein elevations in Crohn's disease. Inflammatory Bowel Diseases. 2018;**24**:2048-2052

[77] Barsky M, Meserve J, Le H, Collins A, Singh S, Boland B, et al. Understanding determinants of patient preferences between stool tests and colonoscopy for the assessment of disease activity in inflammatory bowel disease. Digestive Diseases and Sciences. 2021;**66**(8):2564-2569. DOI: 10.1007/s10620-020-06568-w

Chapter 3

Differential Diagnosis of Ulcerative Colitis

César Enrique Garnica Camacho

Abstract

Nowadays, ulcerative colitis is a diagnostic challenge. It is characterized by being a chronic inflammatory disease that manifests itself with abdominal pain, diarrhea, and hematochezia, associated with an increase in inflammatory markers. In addition, progressive anemia and hypoalbuminemia are found in laboratory tests. The onset of symptoms can be sudden or gradual. Due to not having specific manifestations, the approach can be difficult. Classically, Crohn's disease is a diagnosis that goes hand in hand with ulcerative colitis, however, there are a wide number of diseases to rule out: Diseases of an infectious nature, malignancy, or some even less thought of, such as collagenous colitis or medication-induced colitis. In order to provide adequate treatment, we have to carry out an accurate approach and exclude the main diagnoses.

Keywords: ulcerative colitis, inflammatory bowel disease, Crohn's disease, colitis, Shiga toxin, dysentery, amoebic

1. Introduction

Ulcerative colitis (UC) is part of the spectrum of inflammatory bowel disease, including Crohn's disease (CD).

It is characterized by a uniform inflammation of the colon mucosa, and is classified according to its distribution into proctitis, left colitis, and extensive colitis. This degree of commitment is what gives us the clinical manifestations [1].

Classically, it manifests with abdominal pain, nausea, vomiting, fever, and bloody diarrhea. This last manifestation is characteristic and can be used as a cardinal point to approach the diagnosis. However, there are various inflammatory and infectious disorders that can manifest in the same way, becoming a diagnostic and therapeutic challenge [1, 2]. For this reason, we must perform a broad battery of clinical and imaging studies to approach a more accurate diagnosis.

The purpose of this chapter is to describe in detail the differential diagnoses of UC.

 IntechOpen

2. Approach

2.1 History and clinical manifestations

When we examine a patient with abdominal pain, fever, and diarrhea, the range of diagnostic possibilities is wide [1, 2]. When the number of stools is high and the volume is low (fractioned stools), they contain pus and/or blood (dysentery), we will consider that it is some type of colitis (**Table 1**). In most cases, the first diagnostic possibility is colitis of infectious origin. The most common causal agents are enteropathogenic bacteria, including Shigella, Salmonella, Campylobacter, *Escherichia coli*, among others [3]. These agents regularly appear in both industrialized and underdeveloped countries, and among travelers. Now, when the scenario is different, such as the hospital setting (*Clostridium difficile*), or in an immunocompromised patient (tuberculosis, histoplasmosis, HIV), we will have to consider other pathogens [3–5].

Colitis of infectious origin usually appears suddenly, after ingesting food that is not well cooked, but with self-limitation of the condition with or without treatment [4]. Regularly, the duration does not exceed 1–2 weeks of evolution [3, 4], being those cases of longer duration, which will make us suspect infection by rare pathogens or, even, conditions of non-infectious origin.

Relevant record such as the presence of diverticula, consumption of non-steroidal anti-inflammatory drugs (mainly aspirin) [6], or other medications (laxatives, immunomodulators, or chemotherapy) [7], cancer patients who received pelvic radiation, as well as patients suffering from systemic diseases (vasculitis with colonic condition: polyarteritis nodosa or systemic lupus erythematosus), they can bring us closer to more specific conditions, helping us give specific treatment [1, 4].

Accompanying symptoms such as weight loss, rectal pain, tenesmus, perianal vesicles, genital ulcers, condylomas, lymphadenopathy, erythema nodosum or reactive arthritis will guide us to other less suspected diagnoses such as sexually transmitted diseases or autoimmune diseases [1, 4, 5].

Among the various diseases that mimic UC, we cannot forget CD, which is also part of the spectrum of inflammatory bowel disease. Both share manifestations such as abdominal pain, fever, and diarrhea, but they may have different clinical characteristics [1, 4, 5, 8]. Malabsorption confers anemia, bruising, night blindness, and hypocalcemia with tetany [1, 8].

Gastrointestinal infections: Salmonella, Shigella, Campylobacter, strains of *E. coli, Clostridium difficile, Entamoeba histolytica, Aeromonas, Vibrio, Cytomegalovirus, Mycobacterium.*
Crohn's disease.
Drug-induced colitis: NSAIDs, laxatives, checkpoint inhibitor.
Ischemic colitis
Colorectal cancer
Radiation colitis
Sexually transmitted disease
Autoimmune disease: Behcet's disease, vasculitis.

Table 1.
Differential diagnosis of ulcerative colitis.

In CD, abdominal pain is limited to the right lower quadrant and around the navel, unlike UC, which is located in the left hemiabdomen. Due to uniform rectal involvement, rectal urgency and tenesmus are typical in UC [1, 8].

UC is a disease that affects the mucosa of the colon, presenting mainly as diarrhea with blood (dysentery) in up to 95% of cases [1, 2, 4, 8, 9]. For this reason, we will consider bloody diarrhea as a pivotal symptom. From this manifestation, the diagnostic possibilities will be addressed.

Now, the next step will be to identify those patients who have bloody diarrhea with acute onset (<14 days), from the cases that last longer [3, 4].

2.2 Stool cultures and markers

When a patient comes to our office with acute bloody diarrhea, the most important diagnostic test is a stool culture to look for bacterial causes [3, 4, 9]. The problem is that the result is not immediate and in 45–70% of these cases, it is not possible to identify etiological agents. The precision of the culture decreases if the sample is obtained after the first 3 days of the onset of symptoms [4].

In these cases, we will use other diagnostic resources, such as markers and/or microbiology studies, including cultures and polymerase chain reaction (PCR) tests on feces [3]. The most commonly used fecal markers are leukocytes, lactoferrin, or measurement of calprotectin levels [1–3, 10].

Leukocytes in feces are an inflammation's marker of the intestinal lumen, and strongly suggest infections by Shigella, Salmonella, or inflammatory bowel disease. When there is proctitis or diffuse colonic inflammation, the number of leukocytes is usually high. On the other hand, when it is a focal inflammation, the number of leukocytes is low or absent [2–4]. The drawback is false negatives that appear due to problems in the transfer or handling of the sample and their consequent destruction. To avoid this disadvantage, we can use fecal lactoferrin, a marker released by neutrophilic granules in response to pathogens such as *Escherichia coli*, Salmonella, Shigella, Streptococcus, including Entamoeba [2–4, 11].

Lactoferrin levels are directly proportional to the flow of neutrophils, so its levels indicate how inflamed the intestinal lumen is and, therefore, a direct correlation has been observed with the presence of fecal leukocytes [12]. For example, lactoferrin levels >0.001 microgram/microliter correlate with >200 neutrophils/microliter, which suggests that higher lactoferrin levels imply more fecal neutrophils, more intestinal inflammation, and greater severity [12–16].

Lactoferrin is a marker of neutrophilic, but not lymphocytic, response. For this reason, it does not usually increase when diarrhea is secondary to a viral infection. This was confirmed by Chen et al. where they reported lactoferrin levels of 11.17 ± 2.73 μg/g in patients with Salmonella diarrhea, 10.32 ± 2.94 μg/g in Campylobacter infections, 2.82 ± 1.27 μg/g in rotavirus infections, and 3.16 ± 1.18 μg/g in norovirus patients [16].

The last marker that we will approach is Calprotectin, a protein released by the neutrophil, measured in fecal samples by enzyme-linked immunosorbent assay (ELISA). This biomarker is related to the degree of intestinal inflammation, but is not specific to any disease [1, 3, 11]. There are a 100 causes of intestinal inflammation, so high levels of calprotectin do not differentiate one from another. Enteropathogenic bacterial infections cause variable elevation of calprotectin, as do cases of UC. In industrialized countries, inflammatory bowel disease can be strongly suspected with calprotectin levels >60–100 μg/mg. However, in countries with a high rate of infectious diarrhea (developing countries), even higher levels must be determined to truly suspect inflammatory bowel disease (>200 μg/mg). What is a fact is that levels within the normal ranges of 10–50 μg/mg (as in the case of irritable bowel syndrome) rule out these alterations [17]. Thus, low levels of fecal calprotectin have <1% chance of having inflammatory bowel disease [1, 2].

Elevations of fecal leukocytes, lactoferrin, and calprotectin are related to colonic inflammation, both of infectious (mainly bacterial) and non-infectious origin, so we can infer that they are not useful to define a precise diagnosis [1–3, 18]. Without underestimating its impact on the management of patients with bloody diarrhea, calprotectin can be used to differentiate organic gastrointestinal disorders (UC, colon cancer, celiac disease, infectious colitis) from merely functional causes, such as irritable bowel syndrome [3, 17, 18]. On the other hand, if infectious causes are suspected, then we may consider PCR study in stool.

2.3 Fecal PCR

In recent years, microbiology has progressed enormously. In the past, we depended solely on the results of fecal culture, which, as mentioned above, have a low yield [3, 4, 19]. Recently, technologies have appeared that have allowed us to more quickly identify pathogens in a short time, and with greater precision. Such is the case of PCR studies of single or multiple identification of pathogens [20].

Currently, there are different diagnostic kits that have expanded the number of pathogens detected, especially with the use of multiplex polymerase chain reaction techniques. One of them is FilmArray GI, which was released by the food and drug administration (FDA) for clinical use, allowing the detection of 22 enteric pathogens (**Table 2**) [21, 22].

These novel techniques detect one or more pathogens with high sensitivity and specificity (>98%) in an average time of 2 hours, unlike cultures that usually take >48 hours. The detection rate can be higher than conventional methods, detecting bacterial, parasitic, and viral agents [20–22].

2.4 Endoscopy

Endoscopic studies will be used when we see the need to directly observe the intestinal mucosa, that is, in those cases where the first studies were not revealing, the first treatment did not help resolve the condition, it is an atypical condition or with a longer duration than expected. It is a diagnostic tool that will help us distinguish between UC, CD, and other forms of colitis [1, 4, 5].

The involvement of the colorectal mucosa in UC and terminal ileum in CD is widely known. Continued involvement, ulcerative lesions, erythema, and friability are typical of UC, unlike CD, which is expressed with patchy aphthous ulcers [1, 4, 8, 23].

Up to one-third of patients with suspected UC and bloody diarrhea are due to infectious colitis [24]. Infectious colitis is characterized by mucosa with patchy petechial hemorrhages, edema, and focal erythema [23]. However, this finding does not tell us which pathogen is the culprit, nor whether it is a superinfection in the bed of an inflammatory bowel disease. However, there are findings that bring us closer to infectious causes, such as the preservation of the crypts, viral inclusions (suggestive of cytomegalovirus or herpes simplex virus type II), presence of granulomas (tuberculosis, intracellular *Mycobacterium avium*, syphilis, or *Chlamydia trachomatis*), or whitish plaques that bleed upon removal (characteristic of *Clostridium difficile* colitis) [4, 23, 25].

	Microorganism
Bacteria	• *Campylobacter* (*jejuni*, *coli*, *upsaliensis*) • *Clostridium difficile* • Enteroaggregative *Escherichia coli* • Enteroinvasive *Escherichia coli* • Enteropathogen *Escherichia coli* • Enterotoxigenic *Escherichia coli* • Shiga toxin-producing *Escherichia coli* • *Plesiomonas shigelloides* • *Salmonella* • *Shigella* • *Vibrio cholerae* • *Vibrio parahaemolyticus* and *Vibrio vulnificus* • *Yersinia enterocolitica*
Virus	• Adenovirus • Astrovirus • Norovirus • Rotavirus A • Sapovirus
Parasites	• *Cryptosporidium* • *Cyclospora cayetanensis* • *Entamoeba histolytica* • *Giardia lamblia*

Table 2.
Multiplex PCR: FilmArray GI.

Multiple drugs have been related to colitis symptoms, mainly non-steroidal anti-inflammatory drugs [6]. Chronic consumption (>3 months) of non-steroidal anti-inflammatory drugs can cause small intestine and colon lesions that can mimic both CD and UC. In the United Kingdom, colitis due to Non-steroidal anti-inflammatory drugs (NSAID) is more common than inflammatory bowel disease. These lesions include erythema and edema, superficial or deep ulcerations, crypt distortion, patchy colitis, and lymphoplasmacytic infiltrate [4, 6]. Finally, ischemic colitis, which mainly occurs among elderly people with cardiovascular risk factors, has endoscopic findings of focal lesions characterized by erythema and edema, compromising the rectosigmoid junction or the splenic flexure. In both drug-induced and ischemic colitis, the rectum is usually preserved [4, 7, 23].

3. Specific causes

To facilitate the approach to colitis, the most representative causes of colitis or bloody diarrhea will be developed in detail, as part of the differential diagnosis of UC. We will divide them into acute and chronic causes.

3.1 Acute causes

The main causes of acute colitis are bacterial. We previously mentioned the *Escherichia coli*, Salmonella, Shigella, and Campylobacter (ESSC) complex as the main cause of acute bloody diarrhea, with up to 5 million cases being reported in the United States [1–4, 26]. There are other important agents such as *Entamoeba histolytica* (this germ tends to become chronic), *Clostridium difficile* (important in a hospital environment), and some others.

3.1.1 ESSC complex

E. coli has six strains of clinical relevance, with two strains mainly causing dysentery (>80% of cases), abdominal pain, and fever. These two strains are Shiga toxin-producing *E. coli* and enteroinvasive *E. coli* [26, 27]. Enteroinvasive E. *coli* has been identified as a cause of endemic dysentery in certain countries in South America and Eastern Europe [3].

The clinical picture is usually self-limiting without the need for specific treatment. In severe cases the clinical spectrum can behave like ischemic colitis (in the elderly) or hemolytic uremic syndrome (in young people <15 years of age and elderly). Diagnosis, in the case of Shiga toxin-producing *E. coli* (serotype O157:H7), can be made with detection by fecal PCR [3, 4, 26, 27]. With new microbiology methods, multiplex PCR in Fecal sampling will help us identify the causative strain of *E. coli* [21, 22].

Salmonella usually affects the small intestine and, in a lower percentage, causes colitis and dysentery, causing around 6% of cases in developing countries, changing drastically to 65% in industrialized countries. This suggests underestimated numbers in developing countries due to a lack of laboratory testing [26]. The clinical picture varies from gastroenteritis with watery diarrhea, fever, and abdominal pain with splenomegaly, to enterocolitis with bloody diarrhea, secondary to erosive lesions in Peyer's patches. Symptoms begin 8–48 hours after eating contaminated food, lasting 3–5 days in patients with gastroenteritis and up to 3 weeks in those with enterocolitis. Endoscopic findings vary depending on the patient's manifestations. In patients with bloody diarrhea, colonoscopy demonstrates mucosal friability, ulcerations, aphthous erosions, and deep fissures, with segmental involvement of the colon [28].

Shigellosis commonly results from ingestion of low doses of some strain of Shigella (flexneri, sonnei, dysenteriae, boydii), through food or water, or through sexual contact. The manifestations are fever, anorexia, and vomiting, with abdominal cramps, tenesmus, and mucoid or bloody diarrhea appearing hours later. The usual clinical course lasts no more than a week [4]. Severe cases, with more than 20 bowel movements, dehydration, malnutrition, and persistent diarrhea, are observed in children and immunocompromised patients [29].

Campylobacter as the cause of bloody diarrhea has a prevalence that ranges between 18% and 42%. In many areas of the United States and some developing countries, it is the leading cause of diarrhea [4, 26]. Gastrointestinal symptoms are clinically indistinguishable from those caused by Salmonella and Shigella. Fever may appear in 90% and bloody diarrhea in more than 50% of infections caused by this pathogen. Symptoms are usually self-limiting without treatment, however, up to 20% of cases can persist for 3 weeks. Those severe cases manifest as appendicitis or toxic megacolon [30]. As it is a self-limiting disease, this pathogen is not usually searched for, but when there is doubt (for example, cases lasting >1 week), stool culture is usually requested, even knowing its low effectiveness, which is why multiplex PCR in feces is more useful. Campylobacter dysentery may require short courses of antibiotics [4, 26].

3.1.2 Other important pathogens

When the usual microorganisms (ESSC complex) are ruled out in a patient with bloody diarrhea, other pathogens such as Yersinia, Vibrio, and *Clostridium difficile* become relevant.

Yersinia is a gram-negative bacterium that is acquired from the consumption of foods derived from pork [5]. It is one of the main bacteria causing diarrhea in developing countries, with variable numbers, ranging between 58% and 64%. It has a predilection for children and young people [26]. It manifests itself as fever, watery, and sometimes bloody diarrhea, lasting up to 3 weeks [4, 5]. Since it has a predilection for the cecum and terminal ileum, the abdominal pain is in the right lower quadrant, behaving like pseudoappendicitis in 40% of cases. Colonoscopy shows aphthous ulcers in the right and left colon, and edema and ulcers are observed in the terminal ileum [4, 5, 26, 30].

The different strains of Vibrio, and mainly *Vibrio parahaemolyticus*, cause low-grade fever, nausea, vomiting, nonspecific abdominal pain, and bloody diarrhea in 7% of some series. It usually lasts 3 days, although it can be prolonged in immunocompromised patients [3, 4, 26, 28].

The pathogens mentioned may have a self-limiting course; however, when the symptoms are severe or last longer than usual, we will rely on colonoscopic studies with histopathology to determine if it is an alternative diagnosis, such as UC.

3.1.3 Clostridium difficile

In hospital settings or in people living in a nursing home, the main cause of bloody diarrhea is *Clostridium difficile*. Typically, these patients received antibiotics, mainly broad-spectrum, as well as other agents such as antineoplastics or immunosuppressants. It can manifest with fulminant colitis, colitis with or without pseudomembranes. It manifests itself with bloody diarrhea (10%), fever, and systemic inflammatory response after 1 week of receiving antibiotics [4, 5, 26]. Acute phase reactants usually rise and the leukocyte count increases. The diagnosis is made through the detection of Toxin A and B. Colonoscopy can demonstrate whitish-yellow pseudomembranes in the colon, and raised plaques on the mucosa, associated with patchy or diffuse erythema. Rectum and distal colon are usually involved and 10% involve proximal colon. In less severe cases, colonoscopy findings are absence of membranes, with diffuse or patchy nonspecific colitis [28]. It is noteworthy that the presence of *Clostridium difficile* can coexist with UC, being part of an exacerbation of this disease [1, 2].

3.1.4 Ischemic colitis

Ischemic colitis usually appears when there is a low-flow scenario. It occurs when colonic blood flow (mainly splenic flexure or rectosigmoid junction) is abruptly compromised. Ischemic colitis manifests quickly (within hours) as severe abdominal pain and rectal bleeding. An abdominal CT scan will show us data suggestive of ischemia. An endoscopic study will reveal erythema, edema, friability, superficial and deep ulcers, and images suggestive of gangrene [4]. The single stripe sign (a single linear ulcer of at least 5 cm long on the axis of the left colon) is indicative of ischemic colitis. The clinical course is limited, but occasionally it can become severe (acute mesenteric ischemia), requiring emergency surgery [5].

3.2 Chronic causes

There are various etiologies of bloody diarrhea associated with fever and abdominal pain that may last longer than expected or be related to chronic diseases such as cancer. Likewise, chronic consumption of certain medications can precipitate these manifestations.

3.2.1 Infections

Infection caused by Aeromonas strains causes diarrhea, mainly in the tropics. They usually behave with self-limited diarrhea and rarely cause bloody diarrhea. These cases can last from more than 2 weeks to more than 3 months [3, 4]. These cases with longer duration are the ones that will suggest alternative diagnoses such as UC. Colonoscopy will be of great help in differentiating these conditions [31].

Amoebiasis is an infection caused by *Entamoeba histolytica* that has a high prevalence throughout the world. It is most prevalent in developing countries (e.g., India, Africa, Central and South America). It can be asymptomatic, and cause liver abscesses or colitis. Intestinal symptoms include abdominal pain, fever, and bloody diarrhea (18–48%) after ingestion of contaminated water or food, as well as after sexual contact between homosexual men [4, 26]. Diarrhea may be mild, but it tends to be intermittent and chronic [4, 5]. The initial diagnostic study is with the identification of trophozoites in feces (risk of false positives due to non-pathogenic species) [4, 32]. Detection by PCR is more accurate. Because amoebiasis colitis can be chronic, it can be confused with UC or CD [32, 33]. In these cases, if it cannot be identified directly, or by PCR study, we will request endoscopy (inflammation and ulcerations of the cecum and colon) with biopsy and histopathology [detection of trophozoites by H-E staining (100%), mild alteration of crypt architecture (62.5%), without abscess formation (100%)] to make the differential diagnosis [4, 5, 34].

Sexually transmitted diseases are great imitators. Sexual practices that include anal contact tend to inoculate some of the most common pathogens such as Neisseria gonorrhea, *Chlamydia trachomatis*, human immunodeficiency virus, *Treponema pallidum*, among others. Regarding T. *pallidum* (syphilis), after an incubation of up to 6 weeks, the genital ulcer will appear. In addition to the characteristic genital ulcers, painful anal ulcers, tenesmus, fecal urgency, and fever may occur. Manifestations such as abdominal pain, nausea, vomiting, and bloody diarrhea cast doubt on the diagnosis of a simple venereal disease and may suggest UC. The diagnosis will be made based on the suspected pathogen and the endoscopic findings show ulcers, aphthous lesions, erosions, erythema with colorectal involvement, or terminal ileus [4, 5].

3.2.2 Cancer

Colorectal cancer is a disease with diverse clinical manifestations. Abdominal pain, rectal bleeding, iron deficiency anemia, and diarrhea are found in the broad clinical spectrum. These four signs and symptoms are considered “red flags” since they usually appear at least 3 months prior to the diagnosis of colorectal cancer [35, 36]. The family history of colorectal cancer, abdominal mass, and weight loss will guide us in seeking the diagnosis. Other neoplasms such as lymphomas or carcinoid tumor can be considered, although cases of bloody diarrhea are rare. Generally, diarrhea is inflammatory (leukocytes, blood and/or pus in stool). Given these findings, colonoscopy will show adenomatous polyps (14.4–37.5%), tumors (8%), and ulcers (10.3%) [37].

On the other hand, those patients with some types of cancer, such as melanoma, lung or kidney cancer, receive drugs known as checkpoint inhibitors, such as ipilimumab, nivolumab, or pembrolizumab. Although they have been shown to increase survival, enterocolitis may appear in 21% of cases. This adverse effect requires drug discontinuation, steroid treatment, and anti-TNF treatment, otherwise, there is a risk of perforation and colectomy. The clinical findings resemble inflammatory bowel disease (bloody diarrhea, abdominal pain, fever, vomiting), and endoscopic findings show severe and diffuse damage, with erythema and ulcerations in 79% of patients [5, 38].

Another treatment used for cancer (gastrointestinal, gynecological, urological) is radiotherapy. Depending on the time and dose of radiation, enteritis or proctitis may occur. Manifestations range from abdominal pain, constipation, incontinence, tenesmus, and bloody diarrhea [4, 23]. These events can be acute (<45 days after the last radiation therapy) or chronic (>45 days after radiation). These are usually short-term events, but when they appear a long time after the last radiation session (they can appear up to 30 years later) and without self-limiting symptoms, we would have to consider alternative diagnoses. In these cases, colonoscopy would demonstrate the involvement of the proximal rectum and distal sigmoid. The typical presentation is fragility, granularity, and telangiectasias of the mucosa. In addition, there may be stenosis [23, 39].

3.2.3 Drug-induced colitis

Drug-induced colitis can manifest as microscopic forms (collagenous and lymphocytic colitis) and macroscopic forms (colonic ischemia) [4, 6]. Microscopic colitis manifests with watery diarrhea with normal colonoscopies. More related drugs are proton pump inhibitors, serotonin reuptake inhibitors, and non-steroidal anti-inflammatory drugs, mainly Asprin, with a 30-fold risk with more than 1 year of use [6, 7]. Regarding induced macroscopic colitis due to drugs (non-steroidal anti-inflammatory drugs are the most common cause), it manifests with sudden abdominal pain with or without bloody diarrhea. Endoscopy findings vary according to severity, from edema, petechial hemorrhages, erythema, erosions, or ulcerations, in segments with clear demarcation. Diaphragm-like stenosis is characteristic of macroscopic colitis caused by non-steroidal anti-inflammatory drugs, which is not present in inflammatory bowel disease [4, 6, 40].

3.3 Crohn's disease

UC and CD are inflammatory bowel diseases. Understanding the clinical, serological, and endoscopic characteristics is a fundamental part of the approach to colitis in general. It will be important to detail each of these characteristics to provide the best care for a patient with abdominal pain, fever, and bloody diarrhea.

3.3.1 Manifestations and serology

Among the various diseases that mimic UC, there is CD, which is also part of the spectrum of inflammatory bowel disease. UC is limited to the colon, while CD can occur anywhere in the gastrointestinal tract (ileum and colon: 35%, colon: 32%, small intestine 28%, gastroduodenal: 5%) [41].

Both share manifestations such as abdominal pain, fever, and diarrhea, however, CD usually presents with perianal (fistulas) and anal canal lesions (stenosis, fissures, ulcers), non-bloody and malabsorptive diarrhea [1, 4, 5, 8]. Malabsorption confers anemia, bruising, night blindness, and hypocalcemia with tetany [8].

In CD, abdominal pain is limited to the right lower quadrant and around the navel, unlike UC located in the left hemiabdomen. Finally, due to uniform rectal involvement, rectal urgency and tenesmus are typical in UC [1, 8].

Extraintestinal manifestations can occur in both entities. Musculoskeletal, ocular, and mucocutaneous are the most common. Ankylosing spondylitis and sacroiliitis occur more frequently in CD, unlike primary biliary cholangitis and pyoderma gangrenosum, which are more common in patients with UC [1, 41, 42].

In addition to the clinical differentiation of these diseases, we can rely on serological markers. In addition to the clinical differentiation of these diseases, we can rely on serological markers as Antibodies such as Anti-Saccharomyces cerevisiae (ASCA) and perinuclear pattern antineutrophil cytoplasmic antibodies (pANCA). pANCA are detected mainly in patients with UC (55% vs. 20%), and ASCA in patients with CD (35–50% vs. 1%). These markers have low sensitivity, but can serve as adjuvants to confirm any of the diagnoses [1, 25].

3.3.2 Endoscopy

The uniform involvement of the rectal and colonic mucosa in UC is widely known, unlike CD, where there is focal and transmural involvement in any area of the gastrointestinal tract, with a certain predilection for the terminal ileum and right colon. UC has the endoscopic and histopathological characteristics of erythema, loss of vascular pattern, tissue friability, crypt distortion, and the formation of small ulcers in a linear or circular arrangement [1, 23]. On the other hand, ulcers, Aphthous and longitudinal lesions surrounded by healthy tissue, skipped lesions, luminal stenosis, perianal lesions, and the cobblestone pattern are part of the presentation of CD (**Table 3**) [1, 4, 8, 25].

Characteristics	**Crohn's disease**	**Ulcerative colitis**
Common site	Terminal ileum	Rectum
Bloody diarrhea	No	Yes
Complications	Bowel strictures, obstruction	Toxic megacolon
Lesion pattern	Asymmetric, discontinuous, focal, and patch	Continuous lesion
Ulceration depth	Transmural	Mucosa
Stricture	Common	Rare
Fistula	Common	No
Cobblestone	Yes	No
Microscopy	Non-caseating granulomas	Crypt abscess

Table 3.
Differential diagnosis between Crohn's disease and ulcerative colitis [1, 23, 25].

DOI: http://dx.doi.org/10.5772/intechopen.1008284

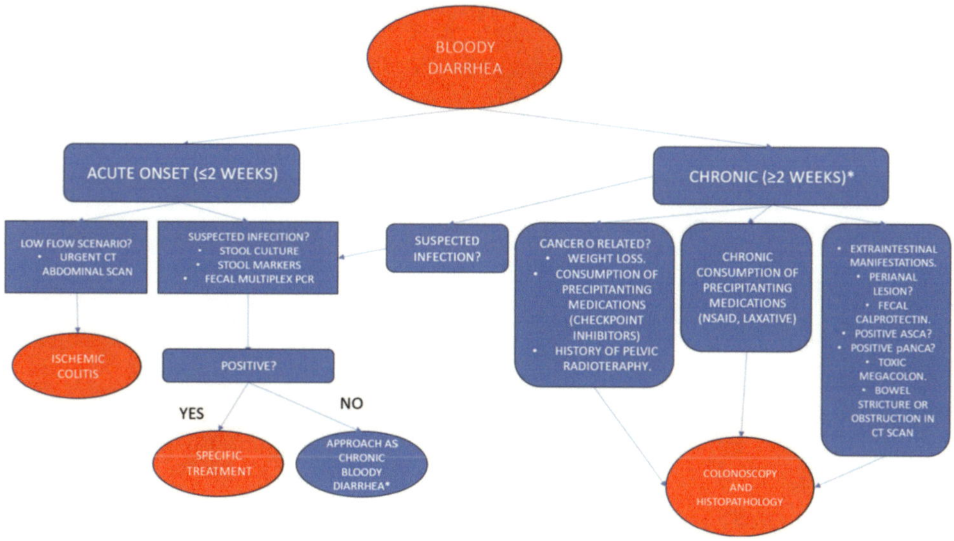

Figure 1.
Differential diagnosis of ulcerative colitis: approach based on bloody diarrhea.

4. Conclusions

When faced with a patient with abdominal pain, fever, and bloody diarrhea of recent onset, we are forced to suspect colitis due to community pathogens, mainly related to the ESSC complex (*E. coli*, Salmonella, Shigella, Campylobacter). Conventional stool cultures will help us confirm these options. If the result is negative, testing for *Clostridium difficile* or *Entamoeba histolytica* may be considered. If we have multiple PCR, we can consider doing it from the first diagnostic approach. Fecal markers such as leukocytes, lactoferrin, or calprotectin can reinforce the initial diagnosis of inflammatory diarrhea, without bringing us closer to a specific diagnosis.

The greatest challenge lies in those patients who present longer, more severe clinical symptoms, or in patients with a significant history of some type of immunocompromise or chronic intake of drugs, such as non-steroidal anti-inflammatory drugs. In these cases, endoscopic studies associated with histopathology will be mandatory (**Figure 1**).

Conflict of interest

The author declares no conflict of interest.

Author details

César Enrique Garnica Camacho
Intensive Care Unit and Internal Medicine Department, General Hospital La Paz, Institute of Security and Social Services of State Workers (ISSSTE), La Paz, Baja California Sur, México

*Address all correspondence to: cesargarnica.mi@hotmail.com

References

[1] Ungaro R, Mehandru S, Allen PB, Peyrin-Biroulet L, Colombel JF. Ulcerative colitis. Lancet. 2017;**389**(10080):1756-1770. DOI: 10.1016/S0140-6736(16)32126-2. Epub 2016 Dec 1

[2] Gros B, Kaplan GG. Ulcerative colitis in adults: A review. Journal of the American Medical Association. 2023;**330**(10):951-965. DOI: 10.1001/jama.2023.15389

[3] DuPont HL. Approach to the patient with infectious colitis. Current Opinion in Gastroenterology. 2012;**28**(1):39-46. DOI: 10.1097/MOG.0b013e32834d3208

[4] Eng SC, Surawicz CM. Differential diagnosis of colitis. Inflammatory Bowel Disease: From Bench to Bedside. 2nd edition. US: Springer; 2003. pp. 431-455. DOI: 10.1007/0-387-25808-6_21

[5] Gecse KB, Vermeire S. Differential diagnosis of inflammatory bowel disease: Imitations and complications. The Lancet Gastroenterology & Hepatology. 2018;**3**(9):644-653. DOI: 10.1016/S2468-1253(18)30159-6. Epub 2018 Aug 8

[6] Geramizadeh B, Taghavi A, Banan B. Clinical, endoscopic and pathologic spectrum of non-steroidal anti-inflammatory drug-induced colitis. Indian Journal of Gastroenterology. 2009;**28**(4):150-153. DOI: 10.1007/s12664-009-0053-9. Epub 2009 Nov 24

[7] Hamdeh S, Micic D, Hanauer S. Drug-induced colitis. Clinical Gastroenterology and Hepatology. 2021;**19**(9):1759-1779. DOI: 10.1016/j.cgh.2020.04.069. Epub 2020 Apr 30

[8] Bernstein CN, Eliakim A, Fedail S, Fried M, Gearry R, Goh KL, et al. World gastroenterology organisation global guidelines inflammatory bowel disease: Update August 2015. Journal of Clinical Gastroenterology. 2016;**50**(10):803-818. DOI: 10.1097/MCG.0000000000000660

[9] Tontini GE, Vecchi M, Pastorelli L, Neurath MF, Neumann H. Differential diagnosis in inflammatory bowel disease colitis: State of the art and future perspectives. World Journal of Gastroenterology. 2015;**21**(1):21-46. DOI: 10.3748/wjg.v21.i1.21

[10] Siciliano V, Nista EC, Rosà T, Brigida M, Franceschi F. Clinical management of infectious diarrhea. Reviews on Recent Clinical Trials. 2020;**15**(4):298-308. DOI: 10.2174/15748871 15666200628144128

[11] Sherwood RA. Faecal markers of gastrointestinal inflammation. Journal of Clinical Pathology. 2012;**65**(11):981-985. DOI: 10.1136/jclinpath-2012-200901. Epub 2012 Jul 19

[12] Abraham BP. Fecal lactoferrin testing. Gastroenterology and Hepatology (New York). 2018;**14**(12):713-716

[13] Lee HM et al. Clinical significance of fecal lactoferrin and multiplex PCR in acute diarrheal disease. Gut and Liver. 2015;**9**(5):636-640. DOI: 10.5009/gnl14106

[14] Mosli MH, Zou G, Garg SK, Feagan SG, MacDonald JK, Chande N, et al. C-reactive protein, fecal calprotectin, and stool lactoferrin for detection of endoscopic activity in symptomatic inflammatory bowel disease patients: A systematic review and meta-analysis. The American Journal of Gastroenterology. 2015;**110**(6):802-819.

quiz 820. DOI: 10.1038/ajg.2015.120. Epub 2015 May 12

[15] Guerrant RL, Araujo V, Soares E, Kotloff K, Lima AA, Cooper WH, et al. Measurement of fecal lactoferrin as a marker of fecal leukocytes. Journal of Clinical Microbiology. 1992;**30**(5):1238-1242. DOI: 10.1128/jcm.30.5.1238-1242.1992

[16] Chen CC, Chang CJ, Lin TY, Lai MW, Chao HC, Kong MS. Usefulness of fecal lactoferrin in predicting and monitoring the clinical severity of infectious diarrhea. World Journal of Gastroenterology. 2011;**17**(37):4218-4224. DOI: 10.3748/wjg.v17.i37.4218

[17] Bjarnason I. The use of fecal calprotectin in inflammatory bowel disease. Gastroenterology and Hepatology (New York). 2017;**13**(1):53-56

[18] Shastri YM, Bergis D, Povse N, Schäfer V, Shastri S, Weindel M, et al. Prospective multicenter study evaluating fecal calprotectin in adult acute bacterial diarrhea. The American Journal of Medicine. 2008;**121**(12):1099-1106. DOI: 10.1016/j.amjmed.2008.06.034

[19] Lee JY, Cho SY, Hwang HSH, Ryu JY, Lee J, Song ID, et al. Diagnostic yield of stool culture and predictive factors for positive culture in patients with diarrheal illness. Medicine (Baltimore). 2017;**96**(30):e7641. DOI: 10.1097/MD.0000000000007641

[20] Garg P, Bhasin SL, Malhotra P, Rana SS, Singh S, Sethi J, et al. Multiplex PCR for gastrointestinal parasites in stool: Benchmarking against direct microscopy and simplex PCR. Diagnostic Microbiology and Infectious Disease. 2024;**110**(2):116475. DOI: 10.1016/j.diagmicrobio.2024.116475. Epub 2024 Jul 30

[21] Hernández RJ, Morales AC, Núñez MM. Impacto de una PCR múltiplex en el diagnóstico y tratamiento en pacientes con gastroenteritis infecciosa. Revista Mexicana de Patología Clínica y Medicina de Laboratorio. 2020;**67**(3):129-141. DOI: 10.35366/96676

[22] Zhang H, Morrison S, Tang YW. Multiplex polymerase chain reaction tests for detection of pathogens associated with gastroenteritis. Clinics in Laboratory Medicine. 2015;**35**(2):461-486. DOI: 10.1016/j.cll.2015.02.006. Epub 2015 Apr 4

[23] Jung SA. Differential diagnosis of inflammatory bowel disease: What is the role of colonoscopy? Clinical Endoscopy. 2012;**45**(3):254-262. DOI: 10.5946/ce.2012.45.3.254. Epub 2012 Aug 22

[24] Tedesco FJ, Hardin RD, Harper RN, Edwards BH. Infectious colitis endoscopically simulating inflammatory bowel disease: A prospective evaluation. Gastrointestinal Endoscopy. 1983;**29**(3):195-197. DOI: 10.1016/s0016-5107(83)72583-6

[25] Lee JM, Lee KM. Endoscopic diagnosis and differentiation of inflammatory bowel disease. Clinical Endoscopy. 2016;**49**(4):370-375. DOI: 10.5946/ce.2016.090. Epub 2016 Jul 29

[26] Pfeiffer ML, DuPont HL, Ochoa TJ. The patient presenting with acute dysentery—A systematic review. The Journal of Infection. 2012;**64**(4):374-386. DOI: 10.1016/j.jinf.2012.01.006. Epub 2012 Jan 13

[27] Gómez-Duarte OG. Enfermedad diarreica aguda por *Escherichia coli* enteropatógenas en Colombia, Acute diarrheal disease caused by enteropathogenic *Escherichia coli* in Colombia. Revista Chilena

de Infectología. 2014;**31**(5):577-586. Spanish. DOI: 10.4067/S0716-10182014000500010

[28] Ina K, Kusugami K, Ohta M. Bacterial hemorrhagic enterocolitis. Journal of Gastroenterology. 2003;**38**(2):111-120. DOI: 10.1007/s005350300019

[29] Kotloff KL, Riddle MS, Platts-Mills JA, Pavlinac P, Zaidi AKM. Shigellosis. Lancet. 2018;**391**(10122):801-812. DOI: 10.1016/S0140-6736(17)33296-8. Epub 2017 Dec 16

[30] Allos BM, Blaser MJ. *Campylobacter jejuni* and the expanding spectrum of related infections. Clinical Infectious Diseases. 1995;**20**(5):1092-1099. quiz 1100-1. DOI: 10.1093/clinids/20.5.1092

[31] Willoughby JM, Rahman AF, Gregory MM. Chronic colitis after Aeromonas infection. Gut. 1989;**30**(5):686-690. DOI: 10.1136/gut.30.5.686

[32] Yakoob J, Abbas Z, Beg MA, Naz S, Khan R, Jafri W. Entamoeba species associated with chronic diarrhoea in Pakistan. Epidemiology and Infection. 2011;**140**(02):323-328. DOI: 10.1017/s0950268811000215

[33] Burgers K, Lindberg B, Bevis ZJ. Chronic diarrhea in adults: Evaluation and differential diagnosis. American Family Physician. 2020;**101**(8):472-480

[34] Yue B, Meng Y, Zhou Y, Zhao H, Wu Y, Zong Y. Characteristics of endoscopic and pathological findings of amebic colitis. BMC Gastroenterology. 2021;**21**(1):367. DOI: 10.1186/s12876-021-01941-z

[35] Fritz CDL, Otegbeye EE, Zong X, Demb J, Nickel KB, Olsen MA, et al. Red-flag signs and symptoms for earlier diagnosis of early-onset colorectal cancer. Journal of the National Cancer Institute. 2023;**115**(8):909-916. DOI: 10.1093/jnci/djad068

[36] Alharbi S, Flemban AF, Kabrah SM, Khogeer AA, Alahmdi H, Mansour AA, et al. The association between colorectal cancer and colonoscopic conditions in Saudi patients: A 10-year cross-sectional-retrospective study. Ethiopian Journal of Health Sciences. 2022;**32**(6):1157-1166. DOI: 10.4314/ejhs.v32i6.13

[37] Abdullah M, Firmansyah MA. Clinical approach and management of chronic diarrhea. Acta Medica Indonesiana. 2013;**45**(2):157-165

[38] Losurdo G, Angelillo D, Favia N, Sergi MC, Di Leo A, Triggiano G, et al. Checkpoint inhibitor-induced colitis: An update. Biomedicines. 2023;**11**(5):1496. DOI: 10.3390/biomedicines11051496

[39] Abu-Sbeih H, Tang T, Ali FS, Ma W, Shatila M, Luo W, et al. Clinical features and management of acute and chronic radiation-induced colitis and proctopathy. Cancers (Basel). 2023;**15**(12):3160. DOI: 10.3390/cancers15123160

[40] Dubeau M-F, Iacucci M, Beck PL, Moran GW, Kaplan GG, Ghosh S, et al. Drug-induced inflammatory bowel disease and IBD-like conditions. Inflammatory Bowel Diseases. 2013;**19**(2):445-456. DOI: 10.1002/ibd.22990

[41] Wilkins T, Jarvis K, Patel J. Diagnosis and management of Crohn's disease. American Family Physician. 2011;**84**(12):1365-1375

[42] Ephgrave K. Extra-intestinal manifestations of Crohn's disease. The Surgical Clinics of North America. 2007;**87**(3):673-680. DOI: 10.1016/j.suc.2007.03.003

Section 2

Management of Ulcerative Colitis

Chapter 4

Use of 5-ASA in Ulcerative Colitis in the Era of Biologics

Ömer Şentürk and Uğur Korkmaz

Abstract

In the era of biologic drugs, 5-aminosalicylic acid (5-ASA compounds) still constitutes the most important step in the treatment of patients with mild-to-moderate ulcerative colitis (UC). They can also be effective at high doses in moderately severe patients who are not at high risk. However, the use of many drugs daily can make it difficult for patients to comply with this group of drugs. Therefore, long-acting, single-dose drugs in the form of the Multi Matrix System (MMX) can play a very important role in treatment management. Although it is not comfortable for every patient, topical 5-ASAs can be used effectively and safely, especially in cases with proctitis and left colon involvement. Mesalazine preparations can also be used safely during pregnancy. In general, the oral dose that provides remission should be the dose selected for maintenance therapy. However, the dose can be reduced over time in topical treatment. Although more robust evidence is needed, 5-ASA preparations are also widely used in the prevention of colorectal cancer (CRC) in UC. 5-ASA drugs have little systemic toxicity. Although safe and well tolerated, patients should still be informed about rare but serious side effects, paradoxical worsening of symptoms at the beginning of treatment, and the need for long-term monitoring of renal function.

Keywords: salazopyrin, sulfasalazine, 5-aminosalicylic acid, mesalazine, mesalamine

1. Introduction

Inflammatory bowel disease (IBD), which occurs as a result of chronic inflammation that cannot be controlled in the intestinal mucosa, manifests itself as two different diseases. Unlike Crohn's disease (CD), which can affect the entire digestive tract from the mouth to the anus and shows full-thickness involvement of the intestinal wall, UC is localized in the large intestine and manifests itself only with mucosa-submucosa involvement and is more common than CD. Although both diseases have common aspects, they show significant differences from pathophysiology to clinical manifestation, from complications to treatment management. The incidence of IBD is increasing with the change in environmental conditions, nutritional habits, and many other factors [1].

New treatment agents (biological agents and small molecules) that emerge every day offer new opportunities to physicians on the one hand, but on the other hand, they bring with them concerns about their limited effects on the course of the disease, potential side effects, and safety. The fact that the desired and expected decrease in surgical colectomy rates has not been demonstrated (at least in some studies) with the introduction of these drugs still makes standard treatments more attractive. In other words, these drugs have limited effects on the course of the disease [2].

The aim of treatment in the disease is to achieve and maintain remission and to maintain quality of life by preventing possible disease-related complications (e.g., cancer, surgery). When deciding on treatment, not only the factors related to the disease, but also the type of medication, dosage, possible side effects, and special conditions of the patient (social status, age, comorbidities, pregnancy status, etc.) should be taken into consideration. For example, steroid side effects may be more important for a young woman or a patient with diabetes. Likewise, the potential malignancy-enhancing effects of immunosuppressive drugs should be considered, especially in young male patients. Similar considerations apply to biological agents. Therefore, physicians should almost always make treatment decisions on a patient-by-patient basis (individualized treatment) [3].

2. Salazopyrin

The discovery of salazopyrin (SASP) or sulfasalazine (sulfasalazine contains 5-aminosalicylic acid that is bound to sulfapyridine *via* a diazo base) in IBD has created a revolutionary effect in the treatment of the disease. Because before SASP, patients were given supportive treatments that were completely symptomatic (bed rest, high protein diet, vitamin supplements, blood transfusion, opioids, and rectal administration of some substances such as bismuth). Undoubtedly, since these treatments had no effect on the disease, the prognosis of the disease was quite poor and mortality was high [4].

The use of SASP, discovered by Nanna Svartz, in patients with UC was reported in a study conducted in 1948 including 124 patients [5]. In this study, it was observed that 80% of mild-moderate UC cases responded to SASP treatment, but almost all of them relapsed when the drug was discontinued. The first double-blind randomized controlled trial (RCT) on SASP was conducted by Baron and colleagues in 1962 [6]. Although SASP given as 4 g was found to be significantly superior to placebo in mild UC cases, many side effects were observed. Subsequently, the same group introduced maintenance therapy by reducing the dose to 2 g and extending the treatment period to 1 year [7]. With this treatment (by extending the treatment period), it was noticed that patients whose treatments had been previously discontinued and who had relapsed in large part remained in remission. This finding was also confirmed in UC patients in whom Dissanayake and Truelove used SASP for 5 years. In this placebo-controlled study, 12% of the placebo group remained in remission, while this rate was found to be 54% in the SASP group ($p < 0.001$). The study concluded for the first time that SASP maintenance treatment of UC should be continued "indefinitely" unless contraindicated due to side effects [8]. As a result, SASP has become the drug of choice worldwide in the treatment of UC.

The prolonged response achieved by reducing the daily dose and prolonging the duration of treatment, as well as increasing the likelihood of potential side effects of the drug, has a serious impact on treatment adherence, prompting new searches for a solution. First, in a placebo-controlled, double-blind study conducted in 1977, it was shown that 5-ASA constitutes the therapeutically active part of sulfasalazine and that sulfapyridine acts as a carrier that allows the release of 5-ASA only in the colon, where the diazo bond is cleaved by bacterial enzymes. Sulfapyridine was found to enter the systemic circulation and was responsible for most of the adverse events associated with sulfasalazine [9]. This situation initiated the process of developing 5-ASA preparations without sulfapyridine.

3. 5-Aminosalicylic acid

There are different forms of 5-ASA. After oral administration, most of the drug is absorbed by the small intestine. The unabsorbed part is excreted in the feces [10]. In order to increase the concentration of 5-ASA in the colonic lumen, different pharmaceutical forms of 5-ASA have been derived, by either time-dependent and pH-dependent or placing it in a matrix (**Table 1**) [11]. The time-dependent release formulation contains microgranules coated with a semipermeable ethyl cellulose membrane. This formulation slowly releases 5-ASA from the duodenum to the ileum in a time-dependent manner, where it is then absorbed by the ileal and colonic mucosa. Therefore, this formulation is used for both UC and CD. In contrast, the pH-dependent release formulation states that 5-ASA is secreted when the threshold pH is exceeded during gastrointestinal transit from the small intestine to the large intestine (pH 6 or 7). When the target pH is reached (e.g., pH > 7), it begins to dissolve in the terminal ileum and shows its effect mainly in the large intestine [12]. Multi-matrix system (MMX) formulations include lipophilic and hydrophilic matrices with Eudragit-S. These coatings release from the terminal ileum and colon at a pH greater than 7, providing an advantage in terms of efficacy and tolerability [13].

5-ASA (mesalamine) is mainly used in IBD due to its anti-inflammatory effects. Although it is not fully understood how it reduces inflammation to date, there are many proposed mechanisms of action since many inflammatory pathways leading to chronic intestinal inflammation have been identified in UC. It achieves its effects by the inhibitory effect it creates on a number of pro-inflammatory substances secreted by the mucosa (**Figure 1**) [14]. Its effect is mainly localized in the area of inflammation and this effect is mainly related to its mucosal concentration. Therefore, the aim when administering this drug should be to ensure that the drug reaches the area of inflammation. For this purpose, the drug can be administered directly into the distal region of the rectum and colon *via* suppository, enema, or foam or orally with different formulations that allow drug distribution into the colon. In fact, when administered as free 5-ASA, the drug is rapidly absorbed and ineffective in the proximal small intestine. Therefore, to achieve the best therapeutic results, it is important to ensure topical availability of the drug on the inflamed mucosa rather than increasing the oral dose [15].

3.1 5-ASA: Use in patients with mild-to-moderate severity

With the discovery of mesalazine and the demonstration of its effectiveness in placebo-controlled studies, the "Mesalazine Era" began in UC. Because before mesalazine, SASP and steroids were drugs with a lot of side effects. Although new drugs that have emerged in the last 10–15 years have reduced the use of mesalazine, it remains the main component of treatment, especially in patients with mild-to-moderate UC. However, the main problem for the physician here is the identification of patients with "Ulcerative Colitis with Mild to Moderate Activity." Because this expression, which is used in all clinical studies demonstrating the effectiveness of mesalazine, has

Formulation	General name	Usage form	Standard daily dose	Place of drug release	Release of the drug	Pharmaceutical technology
Diazo-linked (Azo-linked prodrugs)	Sulfasalazine	Tablet	2–4 g/day	Colon	Cleavage by intestinal flora	5-ASA is linked to sulfapyridine by an azo bond
	Olsalazine	Capsule	2–3 g/day	Colon	Cleavage by intestinal flora	Two 5-ASAs are linked by an azo bond
	Balsalazide	Tablet	2–6.75 g/day	Colon	Cleavage by intestinal flora	5-ASA is linked to 4-aminobenzoyl-b-alanine by an azo bond
Multi-matrix system	MMX mesalamine	Tablet	2.4–3.6 g/day	Terminal ileum, colon	Enteric coated tablet, pH ≥ 7 soluble	MMX is characterized by a lipophilic matrix dispersed within a hydrophilic structure
pH dependent	Mesalamine	Tablet	2.4–4.8 g/day (multiple doses daily)	Terminal ileum, colon	Delayed; pH > 7	Mesalamine is coated with Eudragit S resin
	Mesalamine	Tablet	2.4–4.8 g/day (single daily dose)	Terminal ileum, colon	Delayed; pH > 6–7	Coated with Mesalamine Eudragit L&S resin or natural effective hydrophilic matrix technology
Time dependent	Mesalamine	Tablet, granule, and sachet	2–4 g/day, can be given once a day	From duodenum to colon	Controlled	Ethylcellulose-coated microgranules
Topical	Mesalamine	Enema, foam, and suppository	250 mg–4 g/day	Distal colon and rectum	Topical	Enema, foam, and suppository

Table 1.
5-ASA formulations, release mechanisms, and usage doses. (MMX: Multi MatriX system).

unfortunately not been standardized and the physician's subjective assessment is also included in this calculation [16]. In all studies, the mesalazine group was composed of "Mild-Moderate Activity Ulcerative Colitis" patients, but completely different indexes (with different evaluation criteria) were used in the selection of this group of patients: Clinical Activity Index, Disease Activity Index, Endoscopic Index, Mayo Clinic Endoscopic Subscale, Mayo Clinic Score, Mayo Endoscopic Score, Modified Mayo Disease Activity Index, Patient Functional Assessment, Physician Global Assessment, and Ulcerative Colitis Disease Activity Index.

In determining the appropriate treatment, many factors such as the patient's age, fertility status, additional diseases, and medications taken should be taken into consideration before treatment, in addition to this subjective assessment. In order to

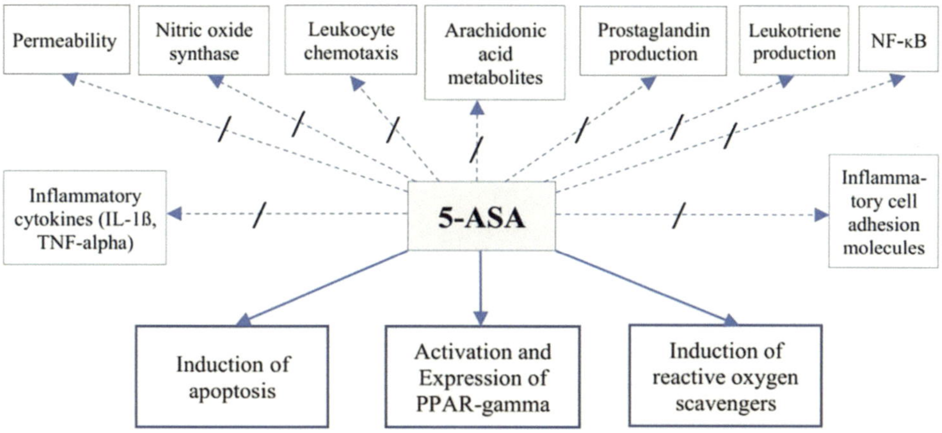

Figure 1.
5-ASA mechanism of action (⊣: inhibitory effect, → stimulatory effect). (IL-1β: Interleukin-1 beta; TNF-alpha: Tumor necrosis factor-alpha; NF-κB: Nuclear Factor kappa B; PPAR-gamma: Peroxisome proliferator-activated receptor).

provide a source for this chapter, we will first explain the use of mesalazine in "Mild-Moderate Activity UC" patients, and then its use in "Moderate Activity UC" patients, which should actually be considered as a separate group. The treatment algorithm for both groups is summarized in **Figure 2**.

Many studies have shown that both oral and topical forms of mesalazine are effective in achieving and maintaining steroid-free remission. One of the first studies on oral 5-ASA was conducted with Asacol®. In patients with mild-to-moderate UC, 4.8 g of Asacol per day was found to produce a higher response rate than placebo (24 vs. 5%). In the same study, 1.6 g of Asacol per day was found to have a similar effect to placebo [15]. The small number of patients included in this study reduces the power of the study. In a multicenter placebo-controlled study, it was suggested that a dose of at least 2.4 g/day was required to detect a clinically significant difference ($p = 0.03$) [17]. According to data from randomized controlled trials, 5-ASA use for 6–8 weeks resulted in 60–70% clinical response and 40–70% clinical remission, with similar rates of endoscopic improvement (30–80%) over the same period. Higher doses resulted in higher mucosal healing at week 6 (80 vs. 68%) [18, 19].

It has been shown in meta-analyses that remission is achieved at higher rates with the continuation of treatment with 5-ASA in patients with remission [20]. In patients who achieved remission with Asacol, the relapse rate in patients who continued treatment was 42.4%, while this rate was 65% in the placebo group [17]. In a meta-analysis of 38 studies including 8000 patients with UC in clinical and endoscopic remission, 41% of patients using 5-ASA experienced relapse, while this rate was found to be 58% in the placebo group (relative risk, 0.69; 95% confidence interval [CI], 0.62–0.77) [21]. In this meta-analysis, no difference was found between the different 5-ASA formulations used in the studies in terms of the effectiveness in maintaining remission [21, 22]. On the other hand, a systematic review of 15 studies on mesalamine and budesonide, a steroid, showed that 2.4 g mesalamine daily was as effective as budesonide-MMX and was better tolerated [23].

Patient compliance is very important in rectal 5-ASA use. In particular, topical mesalazine given alone should be prescribed after the patient has accepted it and has sufficient confidence that it can be applied. Topical mesalazine treatment is superior

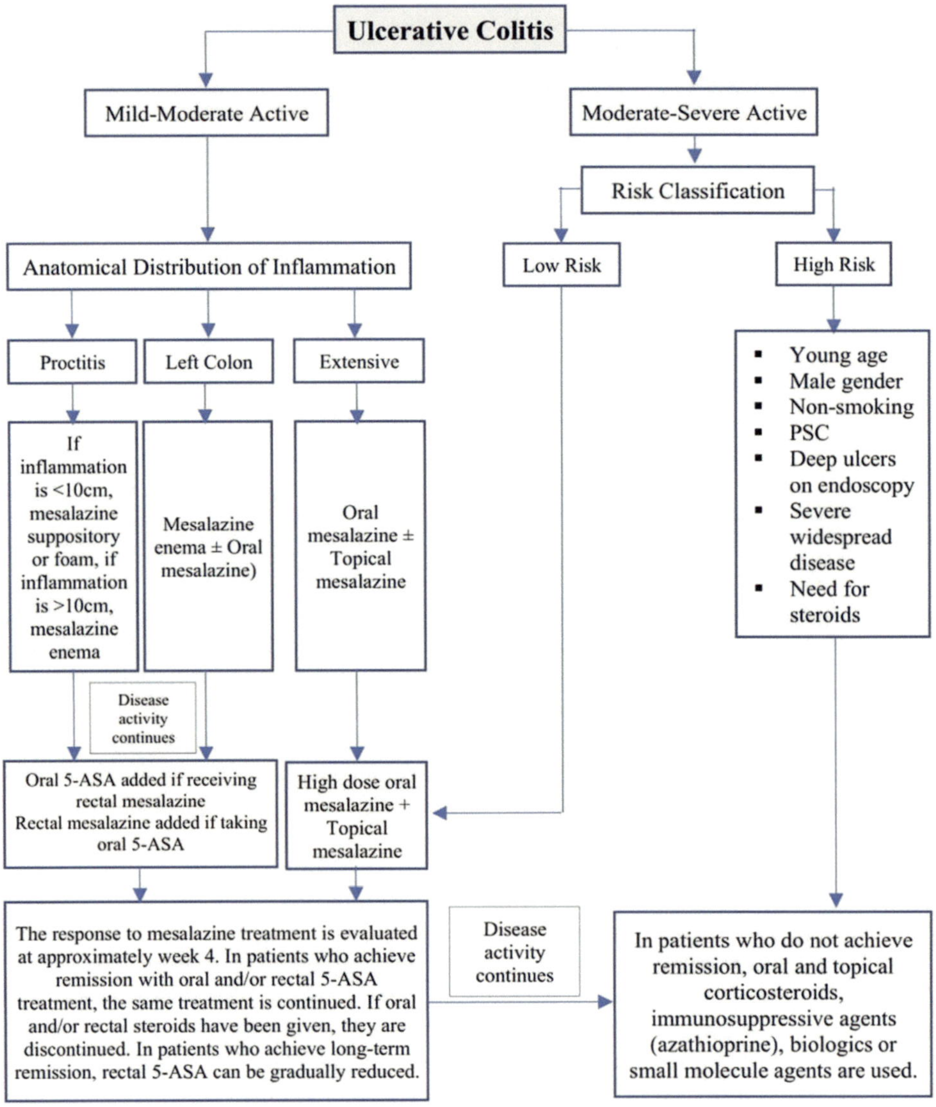

Figure 2.
Algorithm for 5-ASA use in ulcerative colitis. (PSC: Primary sclerosing cholangitis).

to oral 5-ASA in ulcerative proctitis. However, combining topical and oral mesalazine is more effective than topical treatment alone [24] and may protect against the proximal spread of mucosal inflammation in patients with ulcerative proctitis [25]. According to Cochrane systematic reviews, rectal 5-ASA at a dose of 1 g/day is recommended for induction of remission in patients with mild or moderate proctitis to achieve symptomatic, endoscopic, histologic response and remission [26–28]. Suppositories are more suitable for proctitis because they target the rectum better and are better tolerated, but mesalazine foam or enemas can also be used for this indication [29]. Once-daily topical therapy is as effective as divided doses [30]. Topical 5-ASA is more effective than topical steroids alone [31]. However, the combination of topical mesalazine (2 g) and beclomethasone dipropionate (3 mg) has been shown to provide better clinical, endoscopic, and histologic improvement than either agent alone [32]. Topical 5-ASA at a dose of 3 g/week may be sufficient for maintenance treatment of proctitis.

In the treatment of mild-to-moderate left-sided or extensively involved UC, both ECCO and AGA recommend oral mesalazine ≥2 g/day combined with at least 1 g/day of aminosalicylate enemas [26, 27]. This combination strategy has been shown to be more effective than oral 5-ASA alone or topical aminosalicylates alone [33]. There was no difference between foam and liquid enemas in induction of remission [34] or endoscopic healing [35]. Although the optimal duration of combination therapy is uncertain, it has been suggested that daily application for 4 weeks reduces the likelihood of relapse [36].

Topical 5-ASAs are the first choice for maintenance therapy in patients with proctitis after remission induction. However, the frequency of rectal mesalazine use in maintenance of proctitis can be reduced according to the patient's clinical complaints. Rectal mesalazine enemas are a good alternative in left-sided UC [37]. However, the combination of oral and rectal mesalazine has been found to be superior to oral therapy alone or intermittent topical therapy, especially in patients at high risk of relapse [38]. As will be discussed later, new 5-ASA granule formulations [39] and formulations that provide higher levels of 5-ASA in the distal colon, such as MMX-mesalazine [13], may be more effective in this indication.

3.2 Determining the effective dose in 5-ASA treatment

The most important problem facing physicians dealing with UC treatment is the extremely low patient compliance with drug treatment (especially 5-ASA). This is perhaps the most important obstacle to the success achieved with treatment. Patients whose symptoms decrease and/or disappear with 5-ASA treatment either reduce the drug dose, do not take the drug every day, or worse, stop taking the drug. However, a study has unfortunately found that patients who do not comply with 5-ASA maintenance treatment are five times more likely to relapse in the next 2 years compared to patients who comply with the treatment [40]. Here, from the perspective of patients, both frequency and daily 5-ASA intake constitute the main reasons for this incompatibility. Therefore, in order to eliminate this problem, studies have begun to determine the optimum dose of 5-ASA drugs and to develop formulations that provide less frequent daily dosing and lower pill burden.

For mild UC, with fewer than four bowel movements per day, only intermittent bleeding, and no signs of systemic toxicity (fever, tachycardia, anemia, normal erythrocyte sedimentation rate), a starting oral dose of 2.4 g once daily has been found to be as effective as higher doses. For moderate disease (4–6 bowel movements per day, frequent hematochezia, and minimal signs of systemic toxicity), higher doses may provide greater benefit. The 5-ASA dose should be kept high, especially in patients who have previously received systemic corticosteroids. In severe UC (>6 bloody bowel movements per day and significant systemic features), there is no role for 5-ASA [41].

The ASCEND studies in UC are a series of dose-finding studies for 5-ASA. The ASCEND I study investigated oral delayed-release Eudragit S formulation (Asacol®) in divided doses of 4.8 or 2.4 g daily for 6 weeks in patients with mild to moderate UC [42]. The study found no significant difference in achieving overall clinical improvement (i.e., remission or response) between 4.8 and 2.4 g/day of 5-ASA (56 and 51% of patients achieved this primary endpoint, respectively). However, this study found that in the subgroup of patients with moderately active disease, higher therapeutic success was achieved with a higher dose of 5-ASA (72 vs. 57%, $p < 0.05$). The ASCEND II study confirmed that a dose of 4.8 g/day achieved better results than a dose of 2.4 g/day in patients with moderately active UC (72 vs. 59% overall response) [43]. Subgroup analyses of patients with moderate-to-severe UC recruited in the ASCEND III trial showed that a dose of 4.8 g/day was more effective than a dose of 2.4 g/day in patients with a history of difficult-to-treat UC, especially in patients who needed steroids or more than two drugs (steroids, oral 5-ASA, rectal 5-ASA, or immunomodulators) to control their disease in the past [44].

Developed to improved patient compliance with treatment, MMX consists of a lipophilic matrix dispersed in a hydrophilic matrix (double matrix) system. The tablet core contains 5-ASA particles dispersed throughout the hydrophilic matrix within the lipophilic matrix. It is then coated with a polymeric film that is resistant to gastric acid (pH dependent) (allowing the coating to disintegrate at pH ≥ 7.0). This system is designed so that the drug begins to dissolve in the terminal ileum. In a placebo-controlled study on the effect of MMX mesalamine taken once or twice daily for remission induction in patients with mild-to-moderate UC, it was shown that the MMX form was superior to placebo. The study compared MMX 4.8 g/day orally once daily for 8 weeks with 2.4 g/day twice daily 5-ASA (1.2 g PO, given twice daily). Clinical and endoscopic remission was significantly higher in the 5-ASA group compared to placebo (clinical remission 34.1% and endoscopic remission 29.2% in the treatment group and 12.9% in the placebo group, $p < 0.01$). However, there was no significant difference in the responses between the two 5-ASA doses [45]. In a related study, Kamm et al. compared two different doses of MMX 5-ASA given once daily with 2.4 g/day of Eudragit S delayed-release 5-ASA (Asacol®) divided three times daily in patients with mild-to-moderate UC [46]. The primary endpoint of the study, clinical and endoscopic remission rates at 8 weeks were found to be significantly higher in patients receiving MMX mesalamine given as 2.4 g/day once daily (40.5%; $p = 0.01$) and in patients receiving MMX mesalamine given as 4.8 g/day once daily (41.2%; $p = 0.007$), compared to placebo (22.1%).

Subsequently, Sandborn et al. reported analyses combining the patient populations from the above two phase III studies to more precisely estimate the efficacy of MMX mesalazine compared to placebo [13]. In this study, data from a total of 517 patients were analyzed. Eight-week remission rates were 37.2 and 35.1% in the MMX mesalazine 2.4 and 4.8 g/day groups compared with 17.5% in placebo ($p < 0.001$ for both doses compared with placebo). Eight-week complete mucosal healing rates were 32% in both MMX mesalazine groups, compared to 16% in placebo. The incidence of adverse events was similar in all groups. The conclusion was that MMX mesalazine is effective in inducing clinical and endoscopic remission of active, mild-to-moderate ulcerative colitis and is generally well tolerated.

Kamm et al. later reported two phase III studies of MMX in which patients who failed to achieve remission at week 8 continued to receive 5-ASA 4.8 g/day for an additional 8 weeks [47]. These patients were those who had received MMX 2.4 or 4.8 g/day, Asacol 2.4 g/day, or placebo in the main studies. Approximately 60% of patients achieved remission after an additional 8 weeks of MMX 4.8 g/day, regardless of previous therapy. Interestingly, 60% of patients who failed to achieve remission on MMX 4.8 g/day initially achieved remission after an additional 8 weeks of treatment with the same dose of MMX. These findings suggest that 5-ASA treatment can be continued for up to 16 weeks before therapeutic failure is declared. Although this result suggests that essentially equivalent therapeutic success was observed in UC patients after the first 8 weeks of treatment with 2.4 and 4.8 g/day 5-ASA, there may be a reasonable rationale for a step-up approach (i.e., initiating 4.8 g/day 5-ASA in patients who have not achieved therapeutic success after 8 weeks on 2.4 g/day) in patients who receive treatment at 2.4 g/day and do not achieve remission.

In the light of the MMX studies demonstrating the safety, efficacy, and practical advantage of once-daily 5-ASA, other proprietary formulations have been tested. Kruis et al. conducted an equivalence study comparing the once-daily dose of Salofalk® granules (3.0 g/day) with the dose given divided into three daily doses (1.0 g three times daily) in patients with mild-to-moderately active UC [48]. Clinical remission was achieved in 79.1 and 75.7%, respectively, following 8 weeks of once-daily dosing with 3.0 or 1 g three times daily. The only significant difference between the groups was that more patients with proctosigmoiditis achieved remission in the once-daily 5-ASA group. This suggests that the once-daily bolus dose may have achieved higher peak intraluminal concentrations of the drug to better affect inflammation in the distal colon.

Once-daily 5-ASA has been shown to be effective in inducing remission, its efficacy in maintenance has been investigated. Sandborn et al. have shown that 1.6–2.4 g of Asacol once daily is equivalent to twice-daily dosing in preventing UC relapse over a 1-year observation period [49]. Studies of other products have also yielded similar results. Oral ethylcellulose-coated 5-ASA (Pentasa®) has been shown to be statistically superior to the twice-daily 1.0 g format in maintaining clinical remission in UC [50]. The long-term safety and tolerability of MMX 5-ASA at a dose of 2.4 g/day have also been demonstrated [51]. The study also demonstrated that single- or divided-dose MMX regimens were equally effective in maintaining clinical and endoscopic remission in UC for 12 months. MMX 5-ASA at a dose of 2.4 g/day once daily was found to be equivalent to Asacol at a dose of 2.4 g/day twice daily in maintaining clinical remission and mucosal healing for 1 year in patients with left-sided UC [52]. All of the above studies support both the efficacy and safety of the various once-daily dosage formulations of 5-ASA used in the treatment of UC. Clinical trials aside, the new simplified convenient once-daily 5-ASA regimens are likely to be superior to the older 5-ASA multi-dosages in actual clinical practice.

On the other hand, from a safety perspective, aminosalicylates have the best safety profile of all medical therapies currently used in the treatment of IBD. Minor but common side effects of 5-ASA include headache, nausea, indigestion, bloating, and diarrhea. Rare but serious side effects include pleuritis, pericarditis, myocarditis, pancreatitis, and cholestatic hepatitis. Mesalazine-induced nephritis and renal dysfunction have also been described, and it is recommended that renal function be monitored periodically in IBD patients receiving continuous oral 5-ASA maintenance therapy [53]. Patients may experience worsening symptoms of colitis due to the osmotic effects of the drug or, much less commonly, develop eosinophilic colitis with peripheral eosinophilia, characterizing this phenomenon as a drug hypersensitivity reaction.

3.3 5-ASA: Use in moderately severe patients

The majority of clinical evidence for mesalazine has focused on its use in the "Mild to Moderate UC" spectrum, with Cochrane reviews [54, 55] and other meta-analyses [56, 57] confirming its efficacy in both inducing (induction) and maintaining (maintenance) remission in patients with extensive, left-sided, or distal disease. However, in both European and American guidelines, there is a second group of patients defined according to disease activity in determining medical treatment of patients:

"Moderate to Severe UC" [26, 27]. Unfortunately, "Moderate UC" cases in both groups have remained an area of uncertainty and neglect, with the exception of a few studies and one meta-analysis [43, 44, 46, 58].

The definition of moderate disease activity in UC varies in clinical practice and in the medical literature, particularly between early 5-ASA studies and more recent studies evaluating the use of biologics. Randomized controlled trials of 5-ASA compounds [59] included patients with mild-to-moderate UC according to Truelove and Witt's criteria. These patients had: ≤5 bowel movements per day with no more than a small amount of macroscopic blood in the stool, no fever (temperature < 37.8°C), no tachycardia (<90/min), non-severe anemia (>10.5 g/dl), low erythrocyte sedimentation rate (<30 mm per hour) [60]. On the other hand in the study showing the efficacy of infliximab as induction and maintenance therapy in UC [61], the definition of "moderate" disease is different, as eligible patients were those with Mayo score 6–12 [62] and moderate-to-severe active disease at sigmoidoscopy (Mayo endoscopic subscore ≥2) despite concomitant treatment with corticosteroids alone or in combination with thiopurines.

There is currently no formally validated or consensus definition for mild, moderate, or severe UC, but there are three main areas that are important in assessing disease severity in IBD: the impact of the disease on the patient, the burden of disease, and the course of disease [63]. Recently, an expert consensus developed a new index to define overall disease severity by selecting the most important characteristics related to IBD. The disease severity index was generated by accounting for 18.1% of the disease severity being attributed to mucosal lesions, 14.0% to impact on daily activities, 11.2% to C-reactive protein, and 10.1% to previous experience with biologics [64]. The overall disease severity index was then constructed on a 100-point scale by applying the average importance of each attribute to adjusted utilities. Once validated, this disease severity index may provide a useful tool for consistent assessment of overall disease severity in patients with UC.

In fact, at this point, 5-ASA treatment may not be given to all patients with moderate UC, but to selected cases. In this context, if it can be determined which patients and/or disease will have an aggressive course, both at the time of diagnosis and during follow-up, treatment can be established accordingly. Proximal disease extension (left-sided or diffuse colitis) at diagnosis (HR = 1.46, 95% CI = 1.01–2.10, p = 0.04) and baseline hemoglobin level < 10.5 g/dl (HR = 0.43, 95% CI = 0.22–0.81, p = 0.01) were found to be major predictive factors for clinical relapse after 5-ASA/sulfasalazine treatment in patients with mild-to-moderate UC [65]. Two independent predictive factors were identified for the time to relapse after initial oral corticosteroid treatment. Male gender was an unfavorable risk factor (HR = 4, 95% CI = 1.46–11.5, p = 0.03), while long disease duration was found to be a protective factor (HR = 0.98, 95% CI = 0.97–0.99, p = 0.03) [66]. A meta-analysis found that female patients (OR = 0.78, 95% CI = 0.68–0.90) and smokers (OR = 0.55, 95% CI = 0.33–0.91) had a lower risk of colectomy, whereas those with extensive disease (OR = 3.68, 95% CI = 2.39–5.69), those receiving at least one course of corticosteroids (OR = 2.10, 95% CI = 1.05–4.22), and hospitalized patients (OR = 4.13, 95% CI = 3.23–5.27) had a higher risk [67]. In addition to clinical factors, severe endoscopic activity (presence of deep ulcers) and elevated inflammatory markers may also predict an aggressive disease course [27]. On the other hand, concurrent infections (*Cytomegalovirus* or *Clostridium difficile*) increase the risk of disease exacerbation and hospitalization, while primary sclerosing cholangitis (PSC) has been shown to increase the risk of proximal disease spread and CRC [68]. As a result, the "moderate" patient group of

UC can probably be divided into two patient subgroups depending on the presence or absence of these predictors of aggressive disease.

Before determining the treatment of patients, physicians should thoroughly evaluate the findings regarding how the disease may progress and should avoid drugs that have significant side effect potential, especially in repeated or long-term use. On the other hand, this situation should not lead to inadequate treatment in those with severe disease. Unnecessary immunosuppressive treatment should be avoided in a patient whose disease can be managed with 5-ASA. Of course, it may not always be possible to identify this patient group 100%. In addition, there may be no response to the initial 5-ASA, in which case the 5-ASA dose can be increased first by making an individual assessment. In the ASCEND I and II trials, increasing the dose of Asacol® from 2.4 to 4.8 g/day (doubling) in patients with moderate UC led to a significant improvement in clinical efficacy (defined by physician's overall assessment) (58 vs. 72%, $p = 0.04$), with no increase in adverse events [42, 43]. Another study with a different 5-ASA demonstrated the efficacy of high-dose mesalazine (4 vs. 2.25 g/day) in both clinical healing and endoscopic healing. Significant differences were found in all variables used in the UIC disease activity index (UDAI) (stool frequency, rectal bleeding, mucosal appearance on endoscopy) in the high-dose group. In particular, the improvement in mucosal appearance at endoscopy was significantly higher in the high dose group [−0.5 (95% CI = −0.8 to −0.2)] compared to the standard dose group [−0.1 (95% CI = −0.3 to −0.1)] ($p = 0.03$). However, increasing the drug dose did not make a difference in terms of drug reaction or adverse events [69]. This high-dose strategy has also been found to be cost-effective, with high-dose mesalazine being both more effective and less costly than the standard dose [70]. It has also been shown that the addition of topical 5-ASA to this group of patients, in whom the dose of oral mesalazine was increased, reduced the number of relapses and the need for steroids ($p < 0.0001$) [71]. In the study by Kamm et al. [46] comparing MMX mesalazine 2.4 and 4.8 g/day in patients with moderately active UC (placebo-controlled randomized double-blind double-blind, plus 3 equal doses of Asacol® 2.4 g/day in the reference arm), both doses produced higher clinical and endoscopic remission than placebo at week 8 (40.5%; $p < 0.01$, 41.2%; $f < 0.007$ and 22.1%, respectively). In fact, this study investigated the efficacy of once-daily mesalazine MMX form (2.4 and 4.8 g) compared to 2.4 g/day mesalazine given three times daily. The clinical and endoscopic remission rate in the reference arm was not different from placebo (32.6%; $p = 0.124$).

The ASCEND II and III studies showed an advantage of using higher doses of mesalazine [43, 44]. In patients with moderately active UC, Eudragit-S-coated mesalazine 4.8 g/day had a higher treatment success rate than 2.4 g/day (ASCEND II: 71.8 vs. 59.2%, respectively, $p = 0.036$; ASCEND III: 70.2 vs. 65.5%, respectively, $p = 0.17$). Although clinical and complete remission rates were higher for 4.8 g/dose, significant differences were observed only in clinical remission. Clinically importantly, the duration of cessation of rectal bleeding was shorter in patients receiving 4.8 g/day compared to those receiving 2.4 g/day (9 vs. 16 days, respectively; $p = 0.035$) [43]. The clinical significance of this is that if rectal bleeding does not stop within 10 days with high doses (>4 g) of mesalazine, the patient is likely to be a slow or incomplete responder, and therefore, treatment should be reconsidered at that stage. A recent network meta-analysis in patients with only moderately active UC used data from Kamm et al. and the ASCEND II and III studies. The study reported that MMX mesalazine 4.8 g/day combined with Eudragit-S-coated mesalazine 4.8 g/day had overall similar efficacy in achieving clinical and endoscopic remission [58].

Although limited, the available evidence suggests that mesalazine may be an effective and well-tolerated first-line treatment for patients with moderately active UC. The use of mesalazine may be considered for the treatment of patients with moderately active UC, especially those with newly diagnosed disease or relapse after a long period of remission. To maximize the chance of success of treatment, an optimized oral mesalazine dose of ≥4 g/day (±1 g/day rectal mesalazine for proctitis) should be recommended. For patients who respond to this treatment, the IMPACT study has shown that longer-term treatment with mesalazine 4 g/day for at least 6 months significantly reduces the risk of relapse [72]. If a dose reduction is considered after a prolonged period of remission, guidelines recommend continuing oral mesalazine at a minimum of 2 g/day [27, 73]. For patients who do not respond to mesalazine therapy, switching to more effective oral corticosteroids or other therapies should be considered.

4. Use of 5-ASA in special circumstances

4.1 Pregnancy

As the diagnosis of IBD is often made during childbearing years, the management of the disease in reproductive women requires special attention. The most important point in pregnancy and IBD is that the patient who wishes to conceive has been in remission (deep remission) for at least 6 months or more endoscopically [74]. In pregnancies of patients with UC who are not in remission, not only the management of their disease is difficult, but also the effects on the pregnancy/fetus may adversely affect the process. Premature birth, low birth weight babies, miscarriages, and stillbirths are more common in pregnant women with active disease [75, 76]. While Crohn's disease itself can negatively affect pregnancy, only total colectomy + ileal pouch anastomosis in UC reduces pregnancy [77].

The disease state as well as drug therapies should be chosen carefully during pregnancy and all risks related to the disease and drugs should be shared with the patient. Mesalamine is considered safe in pregnancy as no significant adverse effects on the fetus have been observed in animal and human models [78]. A meta-analysis showed that mesalamine use during pregnancy did not increase the rates of congenital malformations, stillbirth, spontaneous abortion, preterm birth, or low birth weight and that doses of more than 3 g per day were safe [79]. Among mesalamine preparations, the FDA revised the pregnancy category of Asacol to C due to the inactive ingredient dibutyl phthalate (DBP) it contains [80]. The reason for this is that DBP has antiandrogenic effects on the fetus exposed during pregnancy and that it can cause urogenital defects in male babies [81]. However, these effects have not yet been demonstrated in human models. Nevertheless, it is recommended that patients using Asacol switch to another mesalamine at least 3 months before pregnancy and that disease control should be provided before pregnancy [82]. If the patient becomes pregnant while using Asacol, an individual approach should be developed. Another drug that should be considered is Sulfasalazine. Pregnant women using Sulfasalazine should receive 2 g of folic acid supplementation daily [75]. Because sulfasalazine crosses the placenta and can affect folate metabolism and cause neural tube defects. Sulfapyridine is found in breast milk and can cause diarrhea in the newborn during breastfeeding [83]. This problem disappears when the drug is stopped. Another point about sulfasalazine is its negative effects on men (expectant fathers) who use this drug. Sulfasalazine use is associated with oligospermia, abnormal sperm morphology, and decreased sperm motility. All of these effects disappear when the drug is stopped. These effects are probably due to the sulfa moiety, and it is recommended to switch to a different drug at least 4 months before planning a pregnancy [74].

4.2 Elderly patients

UC is increasing in all age groups, including early childhood and the elderly population [84]. Elderly UC patients are defined as those >65 years of age [85]. Similar to symptoms in younger patients, elderly UC patients typically present with abdominal pain, urgency, and bloody diarrhea. There is no significant difference in symptomatic severity between the two groups. However, older UC patients are more likely to have UC with left-sided involvement (compared to isolated proctitis and pancolitis) [86].

Compared to the younger population, the health status of elderly patients is more fragile. Not only because of the additional chronic diseases they have and the drugs used to manage them, but also because of the changes in drug metabolism with age and the possible side effects of these drugs, care should be taken in their management. On the one hand, the increased risk of infection and cancer development associated with immunomodulators and biologics should be taken into account, while on the other hand, complications related to the disease as a result of inadequate treatment put gastroenterologists in a difficult position. Another aspect of the matter is the lack of sufficient data on the course of the disease and the effect of treatment in elderly patients. Therefore, the management of UC in elderly patients should be individualized and preferably carried out by physicians experienced in this field or shaped according to the opinion of these physicians [87].

In general, 5-ASAs are considered safe and effective in the treatment of mild-to-moderate UC, but regular monitoring of renal function and side effects, including interactions of 5-ASA with other drugs such as thiopurines, digoxin, warfarin, and isoniazid, should be closely monitored in elderly patients [88].

In addition to oral mesalazine, topical medications can also be used to treat mild-to-moderate UIC in the elderly, but it should be kept in mind that topical mesalazine may increase the rate of fecal incontinence in elderly patients [89].

4.3 Prevention of colorectal cancer (chemoprevention)

The risk of developing CRC is increased in patients with ulcerative colitis. On the one hand, developments in treatment, discovery of new effective drugs, and on the other hand, more dynamic and closer follow-up of patients and the submission of resistant cases to colectomy have reduced the development of cancer in these patients. While it was previously thought that the development of cancer in colitis was six times higher than in the general population [90], more recent data show that this is 2.4 times higher than average [91]. In a study analyzing population-based data on the subject, it was revealed that the risk of CRC in IBD patients was around 1.3–1.6% after 14–15 years [92]. In fact, the risk of CRC has increased at a similar rate not only in patients with UC but also in CD with colonic involvement. The most important approach to preventing this risk is endoscopic screening programs. Since our topic mainly covers the effects of mesalamine, endoscopic screenings will not be discussed.

For a cancer prevention (chemopreventive) approach to be widely used:

1. effective in preventing cancer,
2. easily applicable,
3. affordable,
4. safe and well tolerated,
5. minimal side effects [93].

Almost all of the evidence on the cancer prevention effect of 5-ASA, which meets all the features except the first item above, has been obtained from retrospective examinations of patients who used 5-ASA compliantly (mostly with UC), and unfortunately, there is no randomized, placebo-controlled study on the subject.

A case-control study conducted by Eaden et al. on 102 patients found that the risk of CRC was reduced by 75% in UC patients who received regular 5-ASA treatment (OR 0.25, 95% CI: 0.13–0.48, $p < 0.00001$) [94]. A nested case-control analysis of 18,969 patients found that those who had received six or more 5-ASA prescriptions in the previous 12 months had a lower risk of CRC [95]. In another case-control study, Rubin et al. applied logistic regression analysis to their data and showed that daily 5-ASA doses of 1.2 g or more reduced the likelihood of developing colorectal cancer or dysplasia by 72% and that the degree of protection was dose-related [96].

Velayos et al. published a meta-analysis of 9 studies including 1932 patients examining the association between the use of aminosalicylates and the development of CRC in patients with long-standing UC [97]. In this retrospective meta-analysis of included studies, 5-ASA use was found to have a preventive effect for CRC, but did not alter the risk of dysplasia.

Since retrospective studies and meta-analyses are limited, biased and have the power to interpret data in the desired direction, they are far from objectively answering the cancer preventive effects of 5-ASA. Only prospective, randomized, placebo-controlled studies can answer this question. However, due to the relative rarity of CRC in UC and the long time it takes to develop, such large and long-term studies are unlikely. Nevertheless, additional information on the chemoprophylactic effects of 5-ASA comes from numerous experimental studies with cell culture or animal models of colon epithelial carcinogenesis, confirming that 5-ASA mechanistically inhibits carcinogenesis [41].

Colon cancer in IBD patients is believed to arise differently from sporadic colon cancer in patients without IBD [92, 93]. Unlike sporadic colon cancers that develop in the setting of adenomatous polyps, cancer in IBD patients may develop from nonpolypoid, dysplastic mucosal changes. Active colon inflammation predisposes to dysplasia and is therefore considered a risk factor for colon cancer in patients with IBD. It is therefore conceivable that controlling inflammation of the colon may reduce this risk. At this point, it is conceivable that at least part of the chemopreventive effect of 5-ASA agents is due to their anti-inflammatory effect.

Indeed, these agents are structurally similar to aspirin, an anti-inflammatory drug that has been shown to reduce the rate of sporadic CRC in individuals without IBD [98]. These mechanisms of action include modulation of cyclooxygenase-2, NFkB activity, and scavenging of reactive oxygen species. In particular, PPAR-gamma, a nuclear receptor that mediates colon inflammation in part through modulation of NFkB, has been shown *in vitro* to play an important role in cell cycle progression and apoptosis independent of its anti-inflammatory effect [99]. In addition to its anti-inflammatory effects, 5-ASA has also been shown to have some distinct and specific antineoplastic effects. For example, 5-ASA reduces the activity of the Wnt/beta-catenin pathway [99]. It is well known that increased activity of this pathway is present in most early CRC.

There are currently no definitive guidelines for the use of 5-ASA agents as chemoprevention for CRC. The available evidence is insufficient to support the use of 5-ASA to reduce the risk of malignancy in all individuals with IBD. These agents can be given to patients at higher risk for colon cancer, such as those with extensive disease, primary sclerosing cholangitis, or a family history of CRC. In the prevention of CRC, which has both a low risk and a long time to develop, control of active disease with appropriate treatment approaches and close follow-up should be the basis instead of routine use of 5-ASA.

5. Use of 5-ASA with other drugs

In patients with UC, it is generally recommended to maintain remission with 5-ASA and not to stop the drug, except for a small group of patients with proctitis who remain in remission for a long time [100]. However, the same guideline does not comment on stopping or continuing 5-ASA in patients using immunomodulators and/or biologics [100]. The use of 5-ASA in patients in remission with immunomodulators and/or biologics has attracted the attention of researchers because, on the one hand, it complicates patient compliance with treatment and leads to increased costs, and on the other hand, it is thought to have preventive effects against colorectal cancer [101]. However, the results obtained from observational studies and meta-analyses are contradictory on this issue [102, 103]. The duration and extent of disease, apart from concurrent PSC and family history of CRC, have been identified as modifiable risk factors for chronically active disease CRC [104]. Therefore, any drug that successfully controls inflammation and maintains endoscopic remission may be considered to reduce the risk of CRC, as observed with long-term thiopurine use [105]. A meta-analysis has shown that mesalazine, especially at doses >1.2 g/day, provides a modest reduction in the risk of CRC (OR = 0.6, 95% CI = 0.4–0.9, p = 0.04). However, these studies are not community-based and are based only on data from referral centers [106]. In this context, it remains unclear whether aminosalicylates have an independent biological chemopreventive effect beyond controlling inflammation.

Although the combination of 5-ASA compounds with thiopurines has been shown to have a synergistic effect on thiopurine therapy by increasing serum 6-TGN levels [107–109], in clinical studies, thiopurines combined with 5-ASA were not found to be more effective than thiopurines alone [110, 111]. Therefore, it seems reasonable to try to stop 5-ASA in patients in remission under thiopurines. Conversely, UC patients who are unresponsive or resistant to standard thiopurine therapy may benefit from the concomitant administration of 5-ASA, which may lead to an increase in 6-TGN levels.

The analyses conducted on the use of 5-ASA compounds with biologic agents and the general opinion resulting from this are that these drugs do not provide an additional, positive effect on the treatment [112–114].

6. Compliance problems encountered in the use of 5-ASA

Taking less than 80% of the required dose is defined as "treatment non-adherence." In this case, the patient may have completely stopped the treatment. Therefore, the term non-adherence to 5-ASA treatment refers to patients who stop the treatment or do not follow the treatment regimen correctly [115, 116]. Studies conducted on large patient groups receiving 5-ASA 2–3 times a day reported that almost 60% of UC patients were non-adherent to the treatment [115, 117]. In fact, this problem is not only related to mesalazine. Studies have shown that 20% of IBD patients using azathioprine (AZA) [118] and 30% of those receiving anti-TNF were non-adherent to the treatment [119, 120].

Unfortunately, the most important cause of disease relapse in UC patients is non-adherence to the treatment (**Table 2**). It has been reported that the disease relapse is five times more common in patients who are noncompliant with treatment [40, 121]. The "patient-physician" relationship plays an important role in compliance with drug treatment. The physician should predict the patient's compliance with the treatment and determine the drug to be given and the method of administration accordingly, in other words, an individualized treatment should be applied. Although rectal mesalazine administration is effective, this treatment should not be recommended to a patient who cannot apply it (especially if, e.g., they have pancolitis). However, the effectiveness and importance of this method of administration should be explained to the patient with proctitis and they should be made to understand it. Similarly, for a patient who has difficulty taking the drug orally three times a day, forms that can be administered once a day should be preferred. Detailed information should be

Patient and disease-related factors	Drug-related factors	Physician-related factors	Other factors
• Not accepting the disease • Not accepting the effectiveness of the treatment • Forgetfulness • Intense work schedule • Male gender • Patient's marital status • Short duration of the disease • Prevalence of the disease • Patient's level of education • The disease is in remission	• Route of use (e.g., rectal application) • Taking too many medications or large amounts daily • Seeing or fearing side effects of medications	• The physician does not have sufficient knowledge and experience about the disease • Not providing sufficient information about the disease • Not providing sufficient trust to the patient • The patient cannot reach their physician when necessary	• The patient does not have social security to buy the medicine • The health system is not developed enough to diagnose, treat, and monitor the disease

Table 2.
Reasons for patient non-adherence to mesalamine treatment.

provided to alleviate the patient's concerns about the drugs, and reducing or stopping the drug due to possible side effects should be prevented. The patient should be informed that the disease being in remission does not mean that the disease has disappeared, that stopping the drug may lead to relapse in a large proportion of patients, and the importance of continuing the treatment while in remission should be emphasized. As mentioned before, another important point in the healthy functioning of the treatment process is to avoid polypharmacy. In this context, 5-ASA should not be given to patients in remission with AZA or anti-TNF. Applying the optimum dose to patients in remission with mesalazine to maintain remission is another important point. The higher doses given during remission induction can be gradually reduced after remission is achieved (likewise, treatment frequency can be reduced in topical treatments). Possible reasons for non-adherence to treatment are summarized in **Table 2**. These possible reasons should be considered separately for each patient and individual solutions should be produced.

7. Is there a difference between mesalamines?

Although 5-ASA group drugs are generally effective, especially in patients with mild-to-moderate UC, not all formulations may have the same effect in each patient. Therefore, in cases where clinical response is not obtained, patient compliance is not achieved (such as taking more than one tablet 3 times a day) and some side effects are observed, the drug may be changed. In fact, in patients who do not have side effects or compliance problems, but only inadequate response, the dose should be increased first. However, this increase should not affect the patient's compliance with the drug (such as too frequent, too much medication). A change in drug may be considered for other reasons (e.g., if there are also concerns about tolerance, especially if the patient is taking sulfasalazine or olsalazine, there may be justification for switching to a different 5-ASA treatment). In fact, the most important question at this point is whether patients who do not respond to one formulation of mesalazine (despite appropriate and adequate dosing) should be switched to an alternative preparation or whether the lack of response to one formulation should be considered as a class effect (i.e., should be switched to a more effective class such as steroids). There are very few studies examining the transition from one oral 5-ASA treatment to another. The few published studies have combined a change in 5-ASA formulation with an increase in dose. Although a small study (nine UC patients), patients with endoscopically active disease despite 12 weeks of treatment with Asacol® 2.4 g/day had a significant reduction in the endoscopic severity of the disease when treated with 12 weeks of Pentasa® 4.0 g/day ($p < 0.05$). However, it should be noted that the drug doses used here were not equal [122]. Another study was conducted due to treatment compliance problems (52%), patient preference (36%), and persistence of symptoms (12%). A total of 363 UC patients were examined in this study. Of these, 130 patients (36%) were offered a change and 87 patients (24%) underwent the procedure. In the second study conducted 6 months after the first pilot study, it was found that 70% of the patients had an improvement in their UC severity score (Walmsley Index) and 30% had no change. No worsening of the UC score was observed in any patient. In the second pilot study conducted 6 months later, it was shown that when patients were switched to once daily mesalazine maintenance treatment: 47% reduction in all hospital visits, 60% reduction in hospital visits due to UC flare, 45% reduction in GP visits, and 50% reduction in steroid courses used. Most patients preferred the once daily dose and

85% stated that they were not aware of alternative dosing regimens. Both pilot studies resulted in significant cost savings [123]. Another study by Motoya et al. reported a retrospective analysis of 46 patients with active UC who were switched from a time-dependent mesalazine formulation (4.0 g/day) to a pH-dependent formulation (3.6 g/day) because of inadequate clinical response [124]. At week 8, 50% of patients achieved clinical remission and had a significant decrease in the Lichtiger clinical activity index.

Although further studies are needed, available data suggest that in patients who do not respond adequately to a particular oral 5-ASA treatment, it may be beneficial to increase the dose and/or switch to another oral 5-ASA formulation. The failure of one formulation should not preclude the future use of the entire drug class. Factors such as patient adherence to treatment, site of disease involvement, and activation should be considered when deciding which strategy to use.

On the other hand, patients with stable disease on a particular mesalazine formulation should not switch preparations as this may compromise disease control. In a retrospective study, Robinson et al. showed that stable patients who switched mesalazine formulations had a 3.5-fold increased risk of relapse compared with those who did not switch [125]. This suggests that mesalazine formulations are not bioequivalent.

8. Stopping 5-ASA and reducing the dose

In placebo-controlled studies on stopping topical 5-ASA use in UC patients who had achieved remission, more relapses were seen in the placebo group (52–85% in the placebo group at 12 months, 91% at 24 months, and 20–48% at 12 months and 55% at 24 months in the group continuing 5-ASA use) [126]. Therefore, stopping topical treatment often leads to relapse. Unfortunately, there are no studies on reducing the dose. However, the target of treatment should be to determine the topical dose that will maintain remission. This situation may vary from patient to patient.

The duration of remission is the determining factor in stopping oral 5-ASA. For example, relapse rates were similar to placebo in those who were discontinued after being proven to be in remission for more than 2 years (26 vs. 18%, $p = 0.35$) [127]. However, patients who were in remission for 1–2 years before discontinuation of 5-ASA had a higher relapse rate than those who continued the drug (49 vs. 23%, $p = 0.035$) [127]. Therefore, in patients under 5-ASA monotherapy, the duration of remission should be taken into account when discontinuing the drug and this period should be at least ≥2 years. In addition to the short duration of remission, being younger than 40 years of age and/or having disseminated disease are important risk factors for relapse. The situation with immunosuppressive drugs and biologics has been discussed previously.

A dose-reduction strategy has been put forward to prevent the increased risk of relapse with discontinuation of 5-ASA monotherapy. By reducing the dose, patient compliance can be improved while also reducing treatment costs. The ECCO guideline for the management of UC states that 2 g/day oral 5-ASA is effective in maintaining remission, while in cases of distal disease, topical treatment of 3 g/week in divided doses may be sufficient [26]. Similarly, a retrospective database study of 4452 patients found no significant difference in the risk of exacerbation between patients treated with low-dose (2.2–2.8 g/day) and high-dose (4.4–4.8 g/day) mesalazine over a mean follow-up of 6 years [128]. On the other hand, another randomized controlled trial found that oral mesalazine alone, 1.2 g/day, was less effective than 2.4 g/day in maintaining remission, especially in patients with a history of more frequent relapses [129]. In a different study, 4.8 g/day oral mesalazine was superior to 2.4 g/day in maintaining remission in patients younger than 40 years of age and/or with disseminated disease [130]. In conclusion, it seems safe to reduce the dose in selected patients, but it seems more appropriate to continue high-dose 5-ASA in patients younger than 40 years of age, those with poor drug compliance or those with disseminated colitis.

9. Conclusion

Despite the introduction of new treatment agents every passing day, mesalamines continue to be the main treatment option for UC since the majority of patients have clinically mild and moderate activity. Although classically mild-to-moderate patients are the main indication, 5-ASA preparations have also been shown to be effective in moderate-to-severe UC in selected cases and at high doses. The treatment response increases with the addition of topical agents to oral formulations. They are quite safe agents and can be used safely in both the elderly and pregnant women. Although it has been shown that adding immunosuppressive agents and biologics does not increase the clinical response, these patients still use 5-ASA preparations widely. Likewise, their cancer prevention effects continue to be debated due to the differences in the results obtained from the studies.

Author contributions

Ömer Şentürk determined the topic, conducted literature review on the topic, wrote the text, and created tables and pictures. *Uğur Korkmaz* checked the text, tables, and pictures, and checked for spelling errors.

Conflict of interest

No conflict of interest was reported by the authors.

Author details

Ömer Şentürk[1*] and Uğur Korkmaz[2]

1 Faculty of Medicine, Department of Gastroenterology, Medical Park Göztepe Hospital, Bahçeşehir University, Istanbul, Turkey

2 Department of Gastroenterology, Lokman Hekim Private Hospital, Istanbul, Turkey

*Address all correspondence to: dromersenturk@yahoo.com

References

[1] Kobayashi T, Siegmund B, Le Berre C, Wei SC, Ferrante M, Shen B, et al. Ulcerative colitis. Nature Reviews. Disease Primers. 2020;**6**(1):74. DOI: DOI. 10.1038/s41572-020-0205-x

[2] Dai N, Haidar O, Askari A, Segal JP. Colectomy rates in ulcerative colitis: A systematic review and meta-analysis. Digestive and Liver Disease. 2023;**55**(1):13-20. DOI: 10.1016/j.dld.2022.08.039

[3] Park J, Cheon JH. Updates on conventional therapies for inflammatory bowel diseases: 5-aminosalicylates, corticosteroids, immunomodulators, and anti-TNF-α. The Korean Journal of Internal Medicine. 2022;**37**(5):895-905. DOI: 10.3904/kjim.2022.132

[4] Caprilli R, Cesarini M, Angelucci E, Frieri G. The long journey of salicylates in ulcerative colitis: The past and the future. Journal of Crohn's & Colitis. 2009;**3**(3):149-156. DOI: 10.1016/j.crohns.2009.05.001

[5] Svartz N. The treatment of 124 cases of ulcerative colitis with salazopyrin. Attempts at desensitization in cases of hypersensitiveness to sulphasalazine. Acta Medica Scandinavica. 1948;**131**(Suppl. 206):465. DOI: 10.1111/j.0954-6820.1948.tb12083.x

[6] Baron TH, Connell AM, Lennard-Jones JE, Jones FA. Sulphasalazine and salicylazosulphadimidine in ulcerative colitis. Lancet. 1962;**1**:1094-1096. DOI: 10.1016/s0140-6736(62)92080-9

[7] Misiewicz JJ, Lennard-Jones JE, Connell AM, Baron JH, Jones FA. Controlled trial of sulphasalazine in maintenance therapy for ulcerative colitis. Lancet. 1965;**285**:185-189. DOI: DOI.org/10.1016/S0140-6736(65)90972-4

[8] Dissanayake AS, Truelove SC. A controlled therapeutic trial of long-term maintenance treatment of ulcerative colitis with sulphasalazine (salazopyrin). Gut. 1973;**14**:923-926. DOI: 10.1136/gut.14.12.923

[9] Azad Khan AK, Piris J, Truelove SC. An experiment to determine the active therapeutic moiety of sulphasalazine. Lancet London England. 1977;**2**:892-895. DOI: 10.1016/s0140-6736(77) 90831-5

[10] Zhou SY, Fleisher D, Pao LH, Winward B, Zimmermann EM. Intestinal metabolism and transport of 5-aminosalicylate. Drug Metabolism and Disposition. 1999;**27**(4):479-485

[11] Lamb CA, Kennedy NA, Raine T, Hendy PA, Smith PJ, Limdi JK, et al. British Society of Gastroenterology consensus guidelines on the management of inflammatory bowel disease in adults. Gut. 2019;**68**(Suppl 3):s1-s106. DOI: 10.1136/gutjnl-2019-318484

[12] Desreumaux P, Ghosh S. Review article: Mode of action and delivery of 5-aminosalicylic acid – New evidence. Alimentary Pharmacology & Therapeutics. 2006;**24**(Suppl. 1):2-9. DOI: 10.1111/j.1365-2036.2006.03069.x

[13] Sandborn WJ, Kamm MA, Lishtenstein GR, Lyne A, Butler T, Joseph RE. MMX multi matrix system mesalazine for the induction of remission in patients with mild-to-moderate ulcerative colitis: A combined analysis of two randomized, double-blind, placebo-controlled trials. Alimentary Pharmacology &

Therapeutics. 2007;**26**(2):205-215. DOI: 10.1111/j.1365-2036.2007.03361.x

[14] Doering J, Begue B, Lentze MJ, Rieux-Laucat F, Goulet O, Schmitz J, et al. Induction of T lymphocyte apoptosis by sulphasalazine in patients with Crohn's disease. Gut. 2004;**53**:1632-1638. DOI: 10.1136/gut.2003.037911

[15] Doherty GA, Peppercorn MA. Update on the role of modified release mesalamine in the management of ulcerative colitis and Crohn's disease. Clinical and Experimental Gastroenterology. 2009;**2**:139-147. DOI: 10.2147/ceg.s6145

[16] Caron B, Jairath V, D'Amico F, Al Awadhi S, Dignass A, Hart AL, et al. International consensus on definition of mild-to-moderate ulcerative colitis disease activity in adult patients. Medicina (Kaunas, Lithuania). 2023;**59**(1):183. DOI: 10.3390/medicina59010183

[17] Sninsky CA, Cort DH, Shanahan F, Powers BJ, Sessions JT, Pruitt RE, et al. Oral mesalamine (Asacol) for mildly to moderately active ulcerative colitis. A multicenter study. Annals of Internal Medicine. 1991;**115**(5):350-355. DOI: 10.7326/0003-4819-115-5-350

[18] Ford AC, Achkar JP, Khan KJ, Kane SV, Talley NJ, Marshall JK, et al. Efficacy of 5-aminosalicylates in ulcerative colitis: Systematic review and meta-analysis. The American Journal of Gastroenterology. 2011;**106**:601-616. DOI: 10.1038/ajg.2011.67

[19] Ford AC, Moayyedi P, Hanauer SB. Ulcerative colitis. BMJ. 2013;**346**:f432. DOI: 10.1136/bmj.f432

[20] Rasmussen SN, Bondesen S, Hvidberg EF, Hansen SH, Binder V, Halskov S, et al. 5-aminosalicylic acid in a slow- release preparation: Bioavailability, plasma level, and excretion in humans. Gastroenterology. 1982;**83**:1062-1070

[21] Chaparro M, Gisber JP. Maintenance therapy options for ulcerative colitis. Expert Opinion on Pharmacotherapy. 2016;**17**(10):1339-1349. DOI: 10.1080/14656566.2016.1187132

[22] Ungaro R, Mehandru S, Allen PB, Peyrin-Biroulet L, Colombel J-F. Ulcerative colitis. Lancet. 2017;**389**(10080):1756-1770. DOI: 10.1016/S0140-6736(16)32126-2

[23] Bonovas S, Nikolopoulos GK, Piovani D, Gonzalez-Lorenzo M, Pantavou K, Lytras T, et al. Comparative assessment of budesonide-MMX and mesalamine in active, mild-to-moderate ulcerative colitis: A systematic review and network meta-analysis. British Journal of Clinical Pharmacology. 2019;**85**:2244-2254. DOI: 10.1111/bcp.14051

[24] Safdi M, DeMicco M, Sninsky C, Banks P, Wruble L, Deren J, et al. A double-blind comparison of oral versus rectal mesalamine versus combination therapy in the treatment of distal ulcerative colitis. The American Journal of Gastroenterology. 1997;**92**:1867-1871

[25] Pica R, Paoluzi OA, Iacopini F, Marcheggiano A, Crispino P, Rivera M, et al. Oral mesalazine (5-ASA) treatment may protect against proximal extension of mucosal inflammation in ulcerative proctitis. Inflammatory Bowel Diseases. 2004;**10**:731-736. DOI: 10.1097/00054725-200411000-00006

[26] Harbord M, Eliakim R, Bettenworth D, Karmiris K, Katsanos K, Kopylov U, et al. Third European evidence-based consensus on diagnosis

and management of ulcerative colitis. Part 2: Current management. Journal of Crohn's & Colitis. 2017;**11**:769-784. DOI: 10.1093/ecco-jcc/jjx009

[27] Ko CW, Singh S, Feuerstein JD, Falck-Ytter C, Falck-Ytter Y, Cross RK, et al. AGA clinical practice guidelines on the management of mild-to-moderate ulcerative colitis. Gastroenterology. 2019;**156**:748-764. DOI: 10.1053/j.gastro.2018.12.009

[28] Marshall JK, Thabane M, Steinhart AH, Newman JR, Ananad A, Irvine EJ. Rectal 5-aminosalicylic acid for induction of remission in ulcerative colitis. Cochrane Database of Systematic Reviews. Jan 2010;**20**(1):CD004115. DOI: 10.1002/14651858.CD004115.pub2

[29] van Bodegraven AA, Boer RO, Lourens J, Tuynman HA, Sindram JW. Distribution of mesalazine enemas in active and quiescent ulcerative colitis. Alimentary Pharmacology & Therapeutics. 1996;**10**:327-332. DOI: 10.1111/j.0953-0673.1996.00327.x

[30] Lamet M. A multicenter, randomized study to evaluate the efficacy and safety of mesalamine suppositories 1 g at bedtime and 500 mg twice daily in patients with active mild- to-moderate ulcerative proctitis. Digestive Diseases and Sciences. 2011;**56**:513-522. DOI: 10.1007/s10620-010-1334-y

[31] Marshall JK, Irvine EJ. Rectal corticosteroids versus alternative treatments in ulcerative colitis: A meta-analysis. Gut. 1997;**40**:775-781. DOI: 10.1136/gut.40.6.775

[32] Mulder CJ, Fockens P, Meijer JW, van der Heide H, Wiltink EH, Tytgat GN. Beclomethasone dipropionate (3 mg) versus 5-aminosalicylic acid (2 g) versus the combination of both (3 mg/2 g) as retention enemas in active ulcerative proctitis. European Journal of Gastroenterology & Hepatology. 1996;**8**:549-553. DOI: 10.1097/00042737-199606000-00010

[33] Ford AC, Khan KJ, Achkar J-P, Moayyedi P. Efficacy of oral vs. topical, or combined oral and topical 5-aminosalicylates, in ulcerative colitis: Systematic review and meta-analysis. The American Journal of Gastroenterology. 2012;**107**:167-176. DOI: 10.1038/ajg.2011.410

[34] Cortot A, Maetz D, Degoutte E, Delette O, Meunier P, Tan G, et al. Mesalamine foam enema versus mesalamine liquid enema in active left-sided ulcerative colitis. The American Journal of Gastroenterology. 2008;**103**:3106-3114. DOI: 10.1111/j.1572-0241.2008.02152.x

[35] Römkens TEH, Kampschreur MT, Drenth JPH, van Oijen MGH, de Jong DJ. High mucosal healing rates in 5- ASA-treated ulcerative colitis patients: Results of a meta-analysis of clinical trials. Inflammatory Bowel Diseases. 2012;**18**:2190-2198. DOI: 10.1002/ibd.22939

[36] Paoluzi P, D'Albasio G, Pera A, Paoluzi OA, Pica R, Cottone M, et al. Oral and topical 5-aminosalicylic acid (mesalazine) in inducing and maintaining remission in mild-moderate relapse of ulcerative colitis: One-year randomised multicentre trial. Digestive and Liver Disease. 2002;**34**(11):787-793. DOI: 10.1016/s1590-8658(02)80072-x

[37] Marshall JK, Thabane M, Steinhart AH, Newman JR, Anand A, Irvine EJ. Rectal 5-aminosalicylic acid for maintenance of remission in ulcerative colitis. Cochrane Database of Systematic Reviews. 2012;**11**:CD004118. DOI: 10.1002/14651858.CD004118.pub2

[38] Yokoyama H, Takagi S, Kuriyama S, Takahashi H, Iwabuchi M, Takahashi S, et al. Effect of weekend 5-aminosalicylic acid (mesalazine) enema as maintenance therapy for ulcerative colitis: Results from a randomized controlled study. Inflammatory Bowel Diseases. 2007;**13**:1115-1120. DOI: 10.1002/ibd.20158

[39] Leifeld L, Pfützer R, Morgenstern J, et al. Mesalazine granules are superior to Eudragit-L-coated mesalazine tablets for induction of remission in distal ulcerative colitis - a pooled analysis. Alimentary Pharmacology & Therapeutics. 2011;**34**:1115-1122. DOI: 10.1111/j.1365-2036.2011.04840.x

[40] Kane S, Huo D, Aikens J, Hanauer S. Medication nonadherence and the outcomes of patients with quiescent ulcerative colitis. The American Journal of Medicine. 2003;**114**:39-43. DOI: 10.1016/s0002-9343(02)01383-9

[41] Williams C, Panaccione R, Ghosh S, Rioux K. Optimizing clinical use of mesalazine (5-aminosalicylic acid) in inflammatory bowel disease. Therapeutic Advances in Gastroenterology. 2011;**4**(4):237-248. DOI: 10.1177/1756283X11405250

[42] Hanauer SB, Sandborn WJ, Dallaire C, Archambault A, Yacyshyn B, Yeh C, et al. Delayed-release oral mesalamine 4.8 g/day (800 mg tablets) compared to 2.4 g/day (400 mg tablets) for the treatment of mildly to moderately active ulcerative colitis: The ASCEND I trial. Canadian Journal of Gastroenterology. 2007;**21**:827-834. DOI: 10.1155/2007/862917

[43] Hanauer SB, Sandborn WJ, Kornbluth A, Katz S, Safdi M, Woogen S, et al. Delayed-release oral mesalamine at 4.8 g/day (800 mg tablet) for the treatment of moderately active ulcerative colitis: The ASCEND II trial. The American Journal of Gastroenterology. 2005;**100**:2478-2485. DOI: 10.1111/j.1572-0241.2005.00248.x

[44] Sandborn WJ, Regula J, Feagan BG, Belousova E, Jojic N, Lukas M, et al. Delayed-release oral mesalamine 4.8 g/day (800-mg tablet) is effective for patients with moderately active ulcerative colitis. Gastroenterology. 2009;**137**:1934-1943. DOI: 10.1053/j.gastro. 2009.08.069

[45] Lichtenstein GR, Kamm MA, Boddu P, Gubergrits N, Lyne A, Butler T, et al. Effect of once- or twice-daily MMX mesalamine (SPD476) for the induction of remission of mild to moderately active ulcerative colitis. Clinical Gastroenterology and Hepatology. 2007;**5**(1):95-102. DOI: 10.1016/j.cgh.2006.10.025

[46] Kamm MA, Sandborn WJ, Gassull M, Schreiber S, Jackowski L, Butler T, et al. Once-daily, high-concentration MMX mesalamine in active ulcerative colitis. Gastroenterology. 2007;**132**:66-75. DOI: 10.1053/j.gastro.2006.10.011

[47] Kamm MA, Lichtenstein GR, Sandborn W, Schreiber S, Lees K, Barrett K, et al. Effect of extended MMX mesalamine therapy for acute, mild-to-moderate ulcerative colitis. Inflammatory Bowel Diseases. 2009;**15**:1-8. DOI: 10.1002/ibd.20580

[48] Kruis W, Kiudelis G, Racz I, Gorelov IA, Pokrotnieks J, Horynski M, et al. Once daily versus three times daily mesalazine granules in active ulcerative colitis: A double-blind, double-dummy, randomised, non-inferiority trial. Gut. 2009;**58**:233-240. DOI: 10.1136/gut.2008.154302

[49] Sandborn WJ, Korzenik J, Lashner B, Leighton JA, Mahadevan U, Marion JF, et al. Once-daily dosing of delayed-release oral mesalamine (400-mg tablet) is as effective as twice-daily dosing for maintenance of remission of ulcerative colitis. Gastroenterology. 2010;**138**(4):1286-1296. DOI: 10.1053/j.gastro.2009.12.054. 1296.e1281-1283

[50] Dignass A, Bokemeyer B, Adamek H, Mross M, Vinter-Jensen L, Borner N, et al. Mesalamine once daily is more effective than twice daily in patients with quiescent ulcerative colitis. Clinical Gastroenterology and Hepatology. 2009;**7**(7):762-769. DOI: 10.1016/j.cgh.2009.04.004

[51] Kamm MA, Lichtenstein GR, Sandborn WJ, Schreiber S, Lees K, Barrett K, et al. Randomised trial of once- or twice-daily MMX mesalazine for maintenance of remission in ulcerative colitis. Gut. 2008;**57**:893-902. DOI: 10.1136/gut.2007.138248

[52] Prantera C, Kohn A, Campieri M, Caprilli R, Cottone M, Pallone F, et al. Clinical trial: Ulcerative colitis maintenance treatment with 5-ASA: A 1-year, randomized multicentre study comparing MMX with Asacol. Alimentary Pharmacology & Therapeutics. 2009;**30**:908-918. DOI: 10.1111/j.1365-2036.2009.04117.x

[53] Patel H, Barr A, Jeejeebhoy KN. Renal effects of long-term treatment with 5-aminosalicylic acid. Canadian Journal of Gastroenterology. 2009;**23**:170-176. DOI: 10.1155/2009/501345

[54] Murray A, Nguyen TM, Parker CE, Feagan BG, MacDonald JK. Oral 5- aminosalicylic acid for induction of remission in ulcerative colitis. Cochrane Database of Systematic Reviews. 2020;**8**:CD000543. DOI: 10.1002/14651858.CD000543

[55] Murray A, Nguyen TM, Parker CE, Feagan BG, MacDonald JK. Oral 5-aminosalicylic acid for maintenance of remission in ulcerative colitis. Cochrane Database of Systematic Reviews. 2020;**8**:CD000544. DOI: 10.1002/14651858.CD000544

[56] Paridaens K, Fullarton JR, Travis SPL. Efficacy and safety of oral Pentasa (prolonged-release mesalazine) in mild-to-moderate ulcerative colitis: A systematic review and meta-analysis. Current Medical Research and Opinion. 2021;**37**:1891-1900. DOI: 10.1080/03007995.2021.1968813

[57] Barberio B, Segal JP, Quraishi MN, Black CJ, Savarino EV, Ford AC. Efficacy of oral, topical, or combined oral and topical 5-aminosalicylates, in ulcerative colitis: Systematic review and network meta-analysis. Journal of Crohn's & Colitis. 2021;**15**:1184-1196. DOI: 10.1093/ecco-jcc/jjab010

[58] Paridaens K, Fullarton JR, Travis SPL. Efficacy of oral prolonged-release mesalazine in moderately active ulcerative colitis. JGH Open. 2023;**7**:516-519. DOI: 10.1002/jgh3.12935

[59] Wang Y, Parker CE, Bhanji T, et al. Oral 5-aminosalicylic acid for induction of remission in ulcerative colitis. Cochrane Database of Systematic Reviews. 2016;**4**:CD000543. DOI: 10.1002/14651858.CD000543.pub4

[60] Truelove SC, Witts LJ. Cortisone in ulcerative colitis; final report on a therapeutic trial. British Medical Journal. 1955;**2**:1041-1048. DOI: 10.1136/bmj.2.4947.1041

[61] Rutgeerts P, Sandborn WJ, Feagan BG, Reinish W, Olson A, Johnns J, et al. Infliximab for induction and maintenance therapy for ulcerative colitis. The New England Journal

of Medicine. 2005;**353**:2462-2476. DOI: 10.1056/NEJMoa050516

[62] Schroeder KW, Tremaine WJ, Ilstrup DM. Coated oral 5-aminosalicylic acid therapy for mildly to moderately active ulcerative colitis. A randomized study. The New England Journal of Medicine. 1987;**317**:1625-1629. DOI: 10.1056/NEJM198712243172603

[63] Peyrin-Biroulet L, Panés J, Sandborn WJ, Vermeire S, Danese S, Feagen BG, et al. Defining disease severity in inflammatory bowel diseases: Current and future directions. Clinical Gastroenterology and Hepatology. 2016;**14**(3):348-354.e17. DOI: 10.1016/j.cgh.2015.06.001

[64] Siegel CA, Whitman CB, Spiegel BMR, Feagen B, Sands B, Loftus EV Jr, et al. Development of an index to define overall disease severity in IBD. Gut. 2018;**67**:244-254. DOI: 10.1136/gutjnl-2016-312648

[65] Lee HJ, Jung ES, Lee JH, Hong SP, Kim TI, Kim WH, et al. Long-term clinical outcomes and factors predictive of relapse after 5-aminosalicylate or sulfasalazine therapy in patients with mild-to-moderate ulcerative colitis. Hepato-Gastroenterology. 2012;**59**:1415-1420. DOI: 10.5754/hge10680

[66] Bello C, Belaiche J, Louis E, Reenaers C. Evolution and predictive factors of relapse in ulcerative colitis patients treated with mesalazine after a first course of corticosteroids. Journal of Crohn's & Colitis. 2011;**5**:196-202. DOI: 10.1016/j.crohns.2010.12.011

[67] Dias CC, Rodrigues PP, da Costa-Pereira A, Magro F. Clinical predictors of colectomy in patients with ulcerative colitis: Systematic review and meta-analysis of cohort studies. Journal of Crohn's & Colitis. 2015;**9**:156-163. DOI: 10.1093/ecco-jcc/jju016

[68] Torres J, Caprioli F, Katsanos KH, Lobaton T, Micic D, Zeroncio M, et al. Predicting outcomes to optimize disease management in inflammatory bowel diseases. Journal of Crohn's & Colitis. 2016;**10**:1385-1394. DOI: 10.1093/ecco-jcc/jjw116

[69] Hiwatashi N, Suzuki Y, Mitsuyama K, Munakata A, Hibi T. Clinical trial: Effects of an oral preparation of mesalazine at 4 g/day on moderately active ulcerative colitis. A phase III parallel-dosing study. Journal of Gastroenterology. 2011;**46**:46-56. DOI: 10.1007/s00535-010-0308-3

[70] Buckland A, Bodger K. The cost-utility of high dose oral mesalazine for moderately active ulcerative colitis. Alimentary Pharmacology & Therapeutics. 2008;**28**:1287-1296. DOI: 10.1111/j.1365-2036.2008.03856.x

[71] Frieri G, Pimpo M, Galletti B, Palumba G, Corrao G, Latella G, et al. Long-term oral plus topical mesalazine in frequently relapsing ulcerative colitis. Digestive and Liver Disease. 2005;**37**(2):92-96. DOI: 10.1016/j.dld.2004.09.017

[72] West R, Russel M, Bodelier A, Kuijvenhoven J, Bruin K, Jansen J, et al. Lower risk of recurrence with a higher induction dose of mesalazine and longer duration of treatment in ulcerative colitis: Results from the Dutch, non-interventional, IMPACT study. Journal of Gastrointestinal and Liver Diseases. 2022;**31**:18-24. DOI: 10.15403/jgld-3927

[73] Raine T, Bonovas S, Burisch J, Kucharzik T, Adamina M, Annese V, et al. ECCO guidelines on therapeutics in ulcerative colitis: Medical treatment.

Journal of Crohn's & Colitis. 2022;**16**:2-17. DOI: 10.1093/ecco-jcc/jjab178

[74] Chibbar R, Moss AC. Mesalamine in the initial therapy of ulcerative colitis. Gastroenterology Clinics of North America. 2020;**49**(4):689-704. DOI: 10.1016/j.gtc.2020.07.002

[75] Gaidos JKJ, Kane SV. Managing IBD therapies in pregnancy. Current Treatment Options in Gastroenterology. 2017;**15**:71-83. DOI: 10.1007/s11938-017-0123-5

[76] Magro F, Giochetti P, Eliakim R, Ardizzone A, Armuzzi A, Barreiro-de Acosta M, et al. Third European evidence based consensus on diagnosis and management of ulcerative colitis. Part 1: Definitions, diagnosis, extra-intestinal manifestations, pregnancy, cancer surveillance, surgery, and ileo-anal pouch disorders. Journal of Crohn's & Colitis. 2017;**11**(6):649-670. DOI: 10.1093/ecco-jcc/jjx008

[77] d'Albasio G, Pacini F, Camarri E, Messori A, Trallori G, Bonanomi AG, et al. Combined therapy with 5-aminosalicylic acid tablets and enemas for maintaining remission in ulcerative colitis: A randomized double-blind study. The American Journal of Gastroenterology. 1997;**92**:1143-1147

[78] Mahadevan U, Kane S. American Gastroenterological Association Institute technical review on the use of gastrointestinal medications in pregnancy. Gastroenterology. 2006;**131**:283-311. DOI: 10.1053/j.gastro.2006.04.049

[79] Rahimi R, Nikfar S, Rezaie A, Abdollahi M. Pregnancy outcome in women with inflammatory bowel disease following exposure to 5-aminosalicylic acid drugs: A meta-analysis. Reproductive Toxicology. 2008;**25**(2):271-275. DOI: 10.1016/j.reprotox.2007.11.010

[80] Ham M, Moss AC. Mesalamine in the treatment and maintenance of remission of ulcerative colitis. Expert Review of Clinical Pharmacology. 2012;**5**(2):113-123. DOI: 10.1586/ecp.12.2

[81] Huang PC, Kuo PL, Chou YY, Lin S-J, Lee C-C. Association between prenatal exposure to phthalates and the health of newborns. Environment International. 2009;**35**:14-20. DOI: 10.1016/j.envint.2008.05.012

[82] Mahadevan U, Robinson C, Bernasko N, Bolannd B, Chambers C, Dubinsky M, et al. Inflammatory bowel disease in pregnancy clinical care pathway: A report form the American gastroenterological association IBD parenthood project working group. Gastroenterology. 2019;**156**:1508-1524. DOI: 10.1053/j.gastro.2018.12.022

[83] Shannahan SE, Erlich JM, Peppercorn MA. Insights into the treatment of inflammatory bowel disease in pregnancy. Therapeutic Advances in Gastroenterology. 2019;**12**:1-15. DOI: 10.1177/1756284819852231

[84] Molodecky NA, Soon IS, Rabi DM, Ghali WA, Ferris M, Chernoff G, et al. Increasing incidence and prevalence of the inflammatory bowel diseases with time, based on systematic review. Gastroenterology. 2012;**142**:46-54. DOI: 10.1053/j.gastro.2011.10.001

[85] Ananthakrishnan AN, McGinley EL, Binion DG. Inflammatory bowel disease in the elderly is associated with worse outcomes: A national study of hospitalizations. Inflammatory Bowel Diseases. 2009;**15**:182-189. DOI: 10.1002/ibd.20628

[86] Sturm A, Maaser C, Mendall M, Karagiannis D, Karatzas P, Ipenburg N, et al. European Crohn's and colitis organisation topical review on IBD in the elderly. Journal of Crohn's & Colitis. 2017;**11**:263-273. DOI: 10.1093/ecco-jcc/jjw188

[87] Zhu M, Ran Z. Clinical characteristics of ulcerative colitis in elderly patients. JGH Open. 2021;**5**(8):849-854. DOI: 10.1002/jgh3.12612

[88] Katz S, Surawicz C, Pardi DS. Management of the elderly patients with inflammatory bowel disease: Practical considerations. Inflammatory Bowel Diseases. 2013;**19**:2257-2272. DOI: 10.1097/MIB.0b013e31828c8536

[89] Ford AC, Khan KJ, Sandborn WJ, Hanauer SB, Moayyedi P. Efficacy of topical 5-aminosalicylates in preventing relapse of quiescent ulcerative colitis: A meta-analysis. Clinical Gastroenterology and Hepatology. 2012;**10**:513-519. DOI: 10.1016/j.cgh.2011.10.043

[90] Jess T, Loftus EV, Velayos FS, Harmsen WS, Zinsmeister AR, Smyrk T, et al. Risk of intestinal cancer in inflammatory bowel disease: A population-based study from Olmsted County, Minnesota. Gastroenterology. 2006;**130**(4):1039-1046. DOI: 10.1053/j.gastro. 2005.12.037

[91] Jess T, Rungoe C, Peyrin-Biroulet L. Risk of colorectal cancer in patients with ulcerative colitis: A meta-analysis of population-based cohort studies. Clinical Gastroenterology and Hepatology. 2012;**10**(6):639-645. DOI: 10.1016/j.cgh.2012.01.010

[92] Jess T, Simonsen J, Jørgensen KT, Pedersen BV, Nielsen NM, Frisch M. Declining risk of colorectal cancer in patients with inflammatory bowel disease over 30 years. Gastroenterology. 2012;**143**(2):375-381. DOI: 10.1053/j.gastro.2012.04.016

[93] Chan EP, Lichtenstein GR. Chemoprevention: Risk reduction with medical therapy of inflammatory bowel disease. Gastroenterology Clinics of North America. 2006;**35**:675-712. DOI: 10.1016/j.gtc.2006.07.003

[94] Eaden J, Abrams K, Ekbom A, Jackson E, Mayberry J. Colorectal cancer prevention in ulcerative colitis: A case-control study. Alimentary Pharmacology & Therapeutics. 2000;**14**(2):145-153. DOI: 10.1046/j.1365-2036.2000.00698.x

[95] van Staa TP, Card T, Logan RF, Leufkens HGM. 5-Aminosalicylate use and colorectal cancer risk in inflammatory bowel disease: A large epidemiological study. Gut. 2005;**54**(11):1573-1578. DOI: 10.1136/gut.2005.070896

[96] Rubin DT, LoSavio A, Yadran N, Huo D, Hanauer SB. Aminosalicylate therapy in the prevention of dysplasia and colorectal cancer in ulcerative colitis. Clinical Gastroenterology and Hepatology. 2006;**4**(11):1346-1350. DOI: 10.1016/j.cgh.2006.08.014

[97] Velayos FS, Terdiman JP, Walsh JM. Effect of 5-Aminosalicylate use on colorectal cancer and dysplasia risk: A systematic review and metaanalysis of observational studies. The American Journal of Gastroenterology. 2005;**100**:1345-1353. DOI: 10.1111/j.1572-0241.2005.41442.x

[98] Asano TK, McLeod RS. Nonsteroidal anti-inflammatory drugs and aspirin for the prevention of colorectal adenomas and cancer: A systematic review. Diseases of the Colon and Rectum. 2004;**47**:665-673. DOI: 10.1007/s10350-003-0111-9

[99] Jiang C, Ting AT, Seed B. PPAR-gamma agonists inhibit production of monocyte inflammatory cytokines. Nature. 1998;**391**:82-86. DOI: 10.1038/34184

[100] Doherty G, Katsanos KH, Burisch J, Allez M, Papamichael K, Stallmach A, et al. European Crohn's and colitis organisation topical review on treatment withdrawal ['exit strategies'] in inflammatory bowel disease. Journal of Crohn's & Colitis. 2018;**12**:17-31. DOI: 10.1093/ecco-jcc/jjx101

[101] Lyakhovich A, Gasche C. Systematic review: Molecular chemoprevention of colorectal malignancy by mesalazine. Alimentary Pharmacology & Therapeutics. 2010;**31**:202-209. DOI: 10.1111/j.1365-2036.2009.04195.x

[102] Bonovas S, Fiorino G, Lytras T, Nikolopoulos G, Peyrin-Biroulet L, Danese S, et al. Systematic review with meta-analysis: Use of 5- aminosalicylates and risk of colorectal neoplasia in patients with inflammatory bowel disease. Alimentary Pharmacology & Therapeutics. 2017;**45**:1179-1192. DOI: 10.1111/apt.14023

[103] Nguyen GC, Gulamhusein A, Bernstein CN. 5-aminosalicylic acid is not protective against colorectal cancer in inflammatory bowel disease: A meta-analysis of non-referral populations. The American Journal of Gastroenterology. 2012;**107**:1298-1304; quiz 1297, 1305. DOI: 10.1038/ajg.2012.198

[104] Dulai PS, Sandborn WJ, Gupta S. Colorectal cancer and dysplasia in inflammatory bowel disease: A review of disease epidemiology, pathophysiology, and management. Cancer Prevention Research (Philadelphia, Pa.). 2016;**9**(12):887-894. DOI: 10.1158/1940-6207.CAPR-16-0124

[105] Lu MJ, Qiu XY, Mao XQ, Li XT, Zhang HJ. Systematic review with meta-analysis: Thiopurines decrease the risk of colorectal neoplasia in patients with inflammatory bowel disease. Alimentary Pharmacology & Therapeutics. 2018;**47**:318-331. DOI: 10.1111/apt.14436

[106] O'Connor A, Packey CD, Akbari M, Moss AC. Mesalamine, but not sulfasalazine, reduces the risk of colorectal neoplasia in patients with inflammatory bowel disease: An agent-specific systematic review and meta-analysis. Inflammatory Bowel Diseases. 2015;**21**:2562-2569. DOI: 10.1097/MIB.0000000000000540

[107] Gilissen LPL, Bierau J, Derijks LJJ, Bos LP, Hooymans PM, van Gennip A, et al. The pharmacokinetic effect of discontinuation of mesalazine on mercaptopurine metabolite levels in inflammatory bowel disease patients. Alimentary Pharmacology & Therapeutics. 2005;**22**:605-611. DOI: 10.1111/j.1365-2036.2005.02630.x

[108] Hande S, Wilson-Rich N, Bousvaros A, Zholudev A, Maurer R, Banks P, et al. 5-aminosalicylate therapy is associated with higher 6-thioguanine levels in adults and children with inflammatory bowel disease in remission on 6-mercaptopurine or azathioprine. Inflammatory Bowel Diseases. 2006;**12**:251-257. DOI: 10.1097/01.MIB.0000206544.05661.9f

[109] de Boer NKH, Wong DR, Jharap B, de Graaf P, Hooymans PM, Mulder CJJ, et al. Dose-dependent influence of 5- aminosalicylates on thiopurine metabolism. The American Journal of Gastroenterology. 2007;**102**:2747-2753. DOI: 10.1111/j.1572-0241.2007.01511.x

[110] Campbell S, Ghosh S. Effective maintenance of inflammatory bowel

disease remission by azathioprine does not require concurrent 5-aminosalicylate therapy. European Journal of Gastroenterology & Hepatology. 2001;**13**:1297-1301. DOI: 10.1097/00042737-200111000-00006

[111] Mantzaris GJ, Sfakianakis M, Archavlis E, Petraki K, Christidou A, Karagiannidis A, et al. A prospective randomized observer- blind 2-year trial of azathioprine monotherapy versus azathioprine and olsalazine for the maintenance of remission of steroid-dependent ulcerative colitis. The American Journal of Gastroenterology. 2004;**99**:1122-1128. DOI: 10.1111/j.1572-0241.2004.11481.x

[112] Roth R, Schreiner P, Rossel J-B, Misselwitz B, Scharl M, Rogler G, et al. P604 biologics with or without a combination with 5-ASA in ulcerative colitis: Frequency of usage and effect on the course of disease in the Swiss IBD-cohort study. Journal of Crohn's & Colitis. 2019;**13**:S418-S418. DOI: 10.1093/ecco-jcc/jjy222.728

[113] Singh S, Proudfoot JA, Dulai PS, Jairath V, Fumery M, Xu R, et al. No benefit of concomitant 5-Aminosalicylates in patients with ulcerative colitis escalated to biologic therapy: Pooled analysis of individual participant data from clinical trials. The American Journal of Gastroenterology. 2018;**113**:1197-1205. DOI: 10.1038/s41395-018-0144-2

[114] Ungaro RC, Limketkai BN, Jensen CB, Allin KH, Agrawal M, Ullman T, et al. Stopping 5-aminosalicylates in patients with ulcerative colitis starting biologic therapy does not increase the risk of adverse clinical outcomes: Analysis of two nationwide population-based cohorts. Gut. 2019;**68**:977-984. DOI: 10.1136/gutjnl-2018-317021

[115] Kane SV, Cohen RD, Aikens JE, Hanauer SB. Prevalence of nonadherence with maintenance mesalamine in quiescent ulcerative colitis. The American Journal of Gastroenterology. 2001;**96**:2929-2933. DOI: 10.1111/j.1572-0241.2001.04683.x

[116] Le Berre C, Roda G, Nedeljkovic M, Danese S, Peyrin-Biroulet L. Modern use of 5-aminosalicylic acid compounds for ulcerative colitis. Expert Opinion on Biological Therapy. 2020;**20**(4):363-378. DOI: 10.1080/14712598.2019.1666101

[117] Loftus EV. A practical perspective on ulcerative colitis: Patients' needs from aminosalicylate therapies. Inflammatory Bowel Diseases. 2006;**12**:1107-1113. DOI: 10.1097/01.mib.0000235831.01682.8d

[118] Goodhand JR, Kamperidis N, Sirwan B, Macken L, Tshuma N, Koodun Y, et al. Factors associated with thiopurine non-adherence in patients with inflammatory bowel disease. Alimentary Pharmacology & Therapeutics. 2013;**38**:1097-1108. DOI: 10.1111/apt.12476

[119] Lopez A, Billioud V, Peyrin-Biroulet C, Peyrin-Biroulet L. Adherence to anti-TNF therapy in inflammatory bowel diseases: A systematic review. Inflammatory Bowel Diseases. 2013;**19**:1528-1533. DOI: 10.1097/MIB.0b013e31828132cb

[120] Vangeli E, Bakhshi S, Baker A, Fisher A, Bucknor D, Mrowietz U, et al. A systematic review of factors associated with non-adherence to treatment for immune-mediated inflammatory diseases. Advances in Therapy. 2015;**32**:983-1028. DOI: 10.1007/s12325-015-0256-7

[121] Khan N, Abbas AM, Bazzano LA, Koleva YN, Krousel-Wood M. Long-term oral mesalazine adherence and the

risk of disease flare in ulcerative colitis: Nationwide 10-year retrospective cohort from the veterans affairs healthcare system. Alimentary Pharmacology & Therapeutics. 2012;**36**:755-764. DOI: 10.1111/apt.12013

[122] Wong JM, Wei SC. Efficacy of pentasa tablets for the treatment of inflammatory bowel disease. Journal of the Formosan Medical Association. 2003;**102**:613-619

[123] Prasher H, Savania P, Jazrawi R. Changing patients with ulcerative colitis to once daily mesalazine improves outcome and reduces cost in primary and secondary care. Journal of Crohn's & Colitis. 2013;**7**:S239-S240. DOI: 10.1016/S1873-9946(13)60592-9

[124] Motoya S, Tanaka H, Miyakawa M, Sakemi R, Nasuno M, Imamura A. Efficacy of switching to pH-dependent release formulation of mesalazine at 3.6 g/day from time-dependent release formulation of mesalazine at 4.0 g/day in patients with ulcerative colitis. In: Proceedings of the 10th congress of ECCO; 18-21 February 2015; Barcelona, Spain. Journal of Crohn's and Colitis. 2015;**9**(Suppl. 1):s319-s320

[125] Robinson A, Hankins M, Wiseman G, Jones M. Maintaining stable symptom control in inflammatory bowel disease: A retrospective analysis of adherence, medication switches and the risk of relapse. Alimentary Pharmacology & Therapeutics. 2013;**38**:531-538. DOI: 10.1111/apt.12396

[126] Hanauer S, Goog L, Goodman M, Pizinger RJ, Strum WB, Lyss C, et al. Long-term use of mesalamine (Rowasa) suppositories in remission maintenance in ulcerative colitis. The American Journal of Gastroenterology. 2000;**95**:1749-1754. DOI: 10.1111/j.1572-0241.2000.02185.x

[127] Ardizzone S, Petrillo M, Imbesi V, Cerutti R, Bollani S, Bianchi PG. Is maintenance therapy always necessary for patients with ulcerative colitis in remission? Alimentary Pharmacology & Therapeutics. 1999;**13**:373-379. DOI: 10.1046/j.1365-2036.1999.00473.x

[128] Khan N, Abbas A, Koleva Y, Bazzano L. Long-term mesalamine maintenance in ulcerative colitis: Which is more important? Adherence or daily dose. Inflammatory Bowel Diseases. 2013;**19**:1123-1129. DOI: 10.1097/MIB.0b013e318280b1b8

[129] Paoluzi OA, Iacopini F, Pica R, Marcheggiano A, Consolazio A, Rivera M, et al. Comparison of two different daily dosages [2.4 vs. 1.2 g] of oral mesalazine in maintenance of re-mission in ulcerative colitis patients: 1-year follow-up study. Alimentary Pharmacology & Therapeutics. 2005;**21**:1111-1119. DOI: 10.1111/j.1365-2036.2005.02458.x

[130] Pica R, Cassieri C, Cocco A, Zippi M, Marcheggiano A, De Nitto D, et al. A randomised trial comparing 4.8 vs. 2.4 g/day of oral mesalazine for maintenance of remission in ulcerative colitis. Digestive and Liver Disease. 2015;**47**:933-937. DOI: 10.1016/j.dld.2015.07.011

Chapter 5

Short- and Long-Term Outcomes of Ileal Pouch Anal Anastomosis versus End Ileostomy after Total Proctocolectomy

Jonathan Hughes, Sarai Krewson, Griffin Bryant and Bethany Malone

Abstract

With improvements in medical management, surgery for ulcerative colitis is becoming less frequent. Multidisciplinary care is essential when selecting patients who would benefit from surgery. The most frequent surgical options with curative intent are total proctocolectomy with end ileostomy or total proctocolectomy with ileal pouch-anal anastomosis. When selecting the appropriate operation for a patient, detailed knowledge of short-term outcomes, long-term outcomes, and pouch function is essential. This chapter details indications for surgery, surgical options, patient factors relevant to surgery selection, and short- and long-term outcomes after total proctocolectomy with end ileostomy and total proctocolectomy with ileal pouch-anal anastomosis.

Keywords: ulcerative colitis, J-pouch, total proctocolectomy, toxic colitis, inflammatory bowel disease, ileal pouch anal anastomosis, indeterminate colitis

1. Introduction

Ulcerative colitis is a form of inflammatory bowel disease that affects the rectum and colon. There were an estimated 5 million cases of ulcerative colitis worldwide in 2023, and the incidence is growing [1]. With the advent of biologic and immunomodulating therapies, response to medical management has improved with a decreased need for surgical intervention. However, surgery is still indicated in certain situations and is curative for true ulcerative colitis. The two main surgical options for ulcerative colitis are total proctocolectomy with ileal pouch anal anastomosis reconstruction or total proctocolectomy with permanent end ileostomy. When selecting the appropriate operation, patient factors as well as outcomes and expectations after surgery are important to consider for overall long-term success.

2. Indications for surgery

While the incidence of ulcerative colitis continues to increase worldwide, surgeries have decreased in large part due to improvements in medical management, earlier disease detection and treatment, the creation of evidence-based protocols, and the increased use of biologic therapy and immunomodulators. Despite the improvements in medical management, approximately 20% of ulcerative colitis patients will require surgery, with a lifetime risk of 4.9%, 11.6%, and 15.6% at 1, 5, and 10 years from diagnosis, respectively [2]. Indications for surgery include fulminant colitis, medically refractory disease, steroid dependence, colorectal malignancy, high-grade dysplasia, or multifocal low-grade dysplasia.

Operations within the first year of diagnosis are significantly more likely to be emergent surgeries due to fulminant colitis. Patients with chronic ulcerative colitis requiring inpatient hospitalization also have a 27% risk of requiring a colectomy on the same admission. Emergent colectomy is associated with higher morbidity, mortality, and ultimately pouchitis or other functional issues of an ileal pouch anal anastomosis [3].

With the array of available treatment options, defining medically refractory disease and subsequently which patients would benefit from surgery can be a nuanced decision. Medical treatment options include aminosalicylates, corticosteroids, immunomodulators, synthetic small molecules, and biologic therapy, which are targeted antibodies. The goal of medical management is mucosal healing, which is determined through surveillance colonoscopy. Selection of medications is determined by disease severity, which is scored based on patient symptoms and endoscopic evaluation of mucosal injury [4]. Medical management also includes risks of opportunistic infections, malignancy, osteoporosis, and psychological disease processes such as depression. Therefore, medical management also includes intensive screening for comorbidities of medications, resistance to treatment options, or development of malignancy, as well as preventive measures such as vaccination [5]. Due to the complexities of ulcerative colitis treatment, the decision to proceed with surgery ideally involves a multidisciplinary discussion with the patient's gastroenterologist, primary care physician, and surgeon. In the age of biologic therapy, failure to improve or worsening of disease severity after trial of two immunomodulators and/or biologics would be a strong indicator to consider surgery as third-line therapy is associated with risks of adverse events, serious infections, or death (23%, 7%, and 1%, respectively) [6].

While steroids are integral to inducing remission in severe ulcerative colitis, the adverse effects of dependence include osteoporosis, hypertension, diabetes, Cushing's syndrome, cataracts, glaucoma, and infections [7]. Adverse events related to corticosteroids are estimated to occur in 55% of inflammatory bowel disease patients treated with prednisolone at dosages of 40 mg/day and 33% of patients treated with budesonide 9 mg/day. These risks are also related to the duration of therapy and increase after 2–3 weeks of treatment [8]. Steroid dependence is defined as patients who require 3 months of total duration of steroids or who relapse and require steroid treatment within 3 months of cessation of steroid therapy [9]. Steroid dependence occurs in 22–36% of patients with ulcerative colitis [10, 11]. As steroids are often used as rescue therapy in either the acute setting or in the failure of response to other drug classes, approximately 15% of inflammatory bowel disease patients report self-medication by using steroids without a prescription, which is associated with other risks such as incorrect diagnosis, delays in medical evaluation and intervention, adverse reactions, drug interactions, or covering disease severity leading to steroid dependence [12]. Out of patients who require surgery, 70% are due to medically refractory ulcerative colitis [13].

People living with ulcerative colitis also have an increased risk of colorectal cancer or dysplasia. Risk factors for the development of colorectal cancer include the extent of colonic involvement as well as the length of disease duration. Patients with a larger amount of involved colon have a higher risk than patients with more localized disease. The cumulative incidence rates of colorectal cancer after diagnosis of ulcerative colitis are 2%, 8%, and 18% after 10 years, 20 years, and 30 years, respectively. Rates also vary by geography, with increased rates in the United States and the United Kingdom compared to other countries [14].

3. Surgical options

Surgical approaches to total proctocolectomy fall into three separate categories based on the number of operations: single-stage, two-stage, or three-stage surgery. Single-stage surgery may either involve a permanent ileostomy or an ileal pouch anal anastomosis reconstruction. The selection of staging surgery often depends on patient risk factors as well as emergent or elective indications for surgery.

In the emergent setting, the most common operation is a total abdominal colectomy with end ileostomy. While leaving a rectal stump does introduce the risk of a leak from the rectal stump, there is no formal anastomosis or difficult pelvic dissection. In the emergent setting, the morbidity and mortality for a total abdominal colectomy are half that of a total proctocolectomy with end ileostomy in spite of the often-tenuous rectal stump [15]. If the patient later desires reconstruction, the operations would include a completion proctectomy with ileal pouch anal anastomosis reconstruction and a diverting loop ileostomy followed by loop ileostomy reversal.

In the elective setting, reconstructive options involve an ileal pouch anal anastomosis reconstruction. The purpose of the ileal pouch anal anastomosis is to mimic and restore the reservoir function of the rectum. Pouch designs include S, J, and W configurations, although there are others described. The most commonly performed configuration, the J-pouch, is depicted in **Figure 1**. The technical aspects of pouch formation are beyond the scope of this chapter. The pouch is then stapled to the anus using a circular stapler placed through the rectal cuff. When comparing short-term function of these three configurations, the J-pouch is associated with a higher frequency of defecation, while the S-pouch configuration is associated with a higher need to intubate the anus in order to initiate a bowel movement [17]. While the difference in frequency of defecation may persist up to 1 year after surgery, when followed for 9 years, there is no statistically significant difference in daily or nocturnal stool frequency [18]. The S-pouch configuration also has an 8 times higher risk of developing surgery-related complications, while the J-pouch has a higher risk of developing chronic antibiotic-refractory pouchitis [19]. Due to the increased efficiency of J-pouch formation, decreased risk of surgical complications, and equivalent long-term function, the J-pouch has by far become the most prevalent reconstruction and will be the reconstruction configuration referenced for the remainder of this chapter when discussing ileal pouch anal anastomosis.

The next branch in surgical selection in the elective setting is whether to perform a single-stage total proctocolectomy with reconstruction without a diverting loop ileostomy or to perform a two-stage procedure. Early reviews have shown no significant

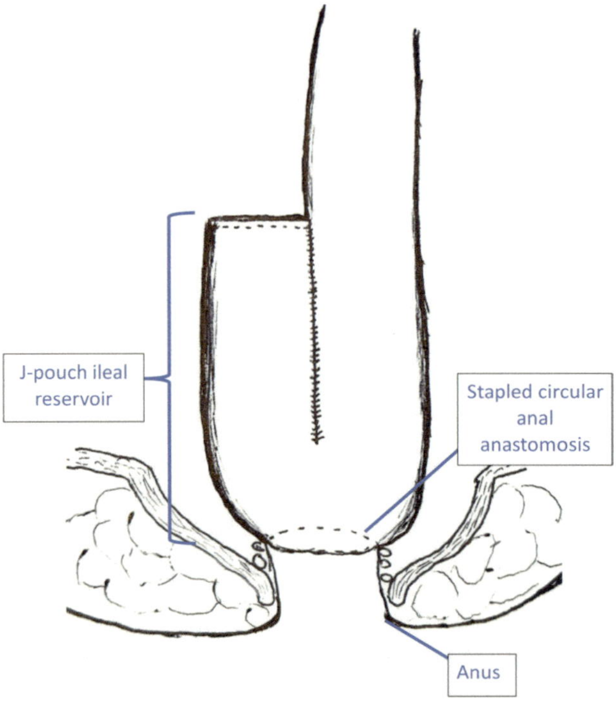

Figure 1.
J-pouch configuration of ileal pouch anal anastomosis Ref. [16].

differences in function when comparing diversion to no diversion. However, diverted patients were more likely to develop small bowel obstructions, and non-diverted or single-stage patients were more likely to develop pelvic sepsis secondary to anastomotic leak [20]. However, with the continued improvement in medical management options as well as increased utilization of minimally invasive techniques such as laparoscopic and robotic-assisted surgery, updated reviews show no statistically significant differences in function or surgical complications but still suggest prudent patient selection for single-stage operations [21]. In a retrospective cohort study performed by Balachandran et al., single-stage proctocolectomy was compared in the elective and emergent settings. While the groups had no significant differences in postoperative complications or function, a subset analysis did show an increased risk of wound dehiscence and pelvic sepsis in patients treated with high-dose preoperative corticosteroids prior to surgery, suggesting that a two-stage operation with a diverting ileostomy should be highly considered in this patient population [22].

While the majority of data has been collected for open operations, the adoption of laparoscopic and robotic-assisted techniques has raised the question as to whether inflammatory bowel disease patients can benefit from a minimally invasive approach. Laparoscopic surgery has been shown to be safe and effective for colorectal surgery with decreased morbidity and length of stay when compared to open procedures [23]. Specifically in surgery for ulcerative colitis, laparoscopic surgery has comparable pouch function to open surgery with decreased morbidity and length of stay [24]. Early data did show significantly increased operative times for laparoscopic versus open surgery, but the difference in operative times vanishes with increased surgeon laparoscopic experience and at high-volume centers [25]. The benefits of the laparoscopic approach are more difficult to prove in the emergent setting, as these patients are more frequently treated by experienced surgeons at high-volume centers. Additionally, these patients do not have the luxury of preoperative optimization of their comorbidities and do not show a decreased length of stay with a laparoscopic versus open approach [26].

The most recent widely adopted advance in minimally invasive colorectal surgery has been robotic-assisted laparoscopic surgery. Robotic surgery does have a lower conversion rate to open surgery when compared to laparoscopic surgery, with a trend but not statistically significant decreased length of stay [27]. Additionally, robotic surgery is associated with a longer surgery duration and higher surgical costs compared to laparoscopic ileal pouch-anal anastomosis [28]. As surgeon expertise in robotic-assisted surgery continues to develop and improve, robotic-assisted surgery has been shown to have decreased short-term outcomes and decreased length of stay compared to laparoscopic surgery for inflammatory bowel disease, while laparoscopic surgery continues to show shorter operative times [29].

4. Short-term outcomes after ileal pouch-anal anastomosis versus end ileostomy

Short-term outcomes refer to items such as length of stay and surgical complications, as long-term pouch and psychosocial function cannot yet be assessed. Both end ileostomy and ileal pouch-anal anastomosis have low mortality rates at approximately 1% within 90 days of surgery [30]. However, these are complex surgeries in complex patients, and morbidity after surgery for ulcerative colitis approaches 40%. Due to the significant risk for associated morbidity, patient comorbidities such as diabetes, frailty, steroid dependence, or cardiopulmonary disease should be considered when choosing between a single procedure with a permanent stoma versus multiple operations [31].

Length of stay is similar between end ileostomy versus ileal pouch-anal anastomosis at an average of 5 days, which is not surprising, as even the J-pouch patients typically have a diverting loop ileostomy, and both groups would require teaching to learn to care for their new stomas [32]. Early operative complications include bleeding, ischemia, anastomotic leak, or pelvic sepsis. While bleeding and ischemia can occur in either operation, the introduced risks of anastomotic leak and pelvic sepsis are introduced through the addition of an ileal pouch-anal anastomosis. Due to the anatomy of the J-pouch, a leak can occur from either the pouch-to-anus anastomosis or from the J-pouch itself, with the most common leak source being the pouch-anal anastomosis. The leak rate after ileal pouch anal anastomosis ranges from 10 to 17% [33].

When comparing laparoscopic versus open approaches, mortality is similar, while length of stay is shorter with a laparoscopic approach. Other benefits of a laparoscopic approach include decreased narcotic use, earlier return of bowel function, and decreased risk of early complications. However, the early complication rate may be confounded by decreased disease severity, which influenced the selection of a laparoscopic approach. Patients who initially underwent laparoscopic total abdominal colectomy with a three-staged reconstruction compared to open total abdominal colectomy had higher serum albumin prior to the index operation (a marker for baseline nutritional status), less inpatient narcotic usage, faster return of bowel function, and shorter length of stay and proceeded with their second and third stages of surgical reconstruction 49 days sooner and 17 days sooner, respectively [34]. As previously discussed, there is little data to support a difference between a laparoscopic and a robotic-assisted surgical approach, but a robotic-assisted approach is associated with longer operative times and a decreased conversion to open surgery [35].

5. Long-term outcomes after ileal pouch-anal anastomosis versus end ileostomy

While ileostomy function does not change with time, the function of a J-pouch can. Both end ileostomy patients and restorative ileal pouch-anal anastomosis patients have high rates of satisfaction, ranging from 80 to 96%. Interestingly, body image concerns are more associated with open surgery compared to minimally invasive surgery and less associated with a permanent ileostomy, with better body image in the minimally invasive surgery group [36]. Quality of life scores regarding social restrictions, performance status, lifestyle satisfaction, ability to return to work or school, body image, and participation in sexual relationships are similar between end ileostomy versus J-pouch patients [37].

Pouchitis is a frequent complication of a J-pouch, which is defined as inflammation of the ileal-anal pouch and occurs in 30–50% of patients. Symptoms can include pain, bleeding, frequency, and urgency. Treatment options include antibiotics or immunosuppressants delivered orally, rectally, or systemically with subcutaneous injections or intravenous infusions, depending on the severity [38]. Approximately 17% of patients will then progress to develop chronic antibiotic-refractory pouchitis, which may become severe enough to warrant pouch excision with conversion to an end ileostomy [39].

Bowel function after J-pouch reconstruction should be discussed with patients preoperatively in order to set appropriate postoperative expectations. On average, most patients experience six to eight loose bowel movements during the day and two bowel movements at night [18, 40]. Urgency, defined as needing to defecate within 15 minutes of having the urge, is another concern after the J-pouch. In severe ulcerative colitis, 41% of patients report fecal urgency. This is similar to fecal urgency within the first year of restorative proctocolectomy with J-pouch reconstruction [41]. However, with appropriate postoperative counseling, physical therapy, stool management, and patient selection, up to 90% of patients can delay defecation over 15 minutes from the urge to defecate [42]. However, 56.4% of patients report needing to have another bowel movement within 15 minutes of a previous bowel movement, and up to 50% report the sensation of incomplete evacuation of stool [43].

Due to the combination of looser stool with fecal urgency, fecal incontinence is another concern for postoperative function after J-pouch reconstruction, and preoperative fecal incontinence is a contraindication for restorative proctocolectomy with ileal pouch-anal anastomosis. With appropriate patient selection, 79–91% of patients report none or seldom incontinent episodes [42]. However, as happens in non-surgical patients, fecal incontinence does increase with age. Comparing function 1 year after J-pouch to 20 years after J-pouch, daytime incontinent episodes increase from 5 to 11%, and nocturnal incontinent episodes increase from 12 to 21% despite no change in the use of stool bulking agents or patient ability to differentiate stool from flatus [44]. In order to combat these issues, 46% of patients report making dietary changes to avoid loose stools and incontinent episodes [45]. Up to 50% of patients report taking antidiarrheal medications in order to combat fecal incontinence [2]. Sacral nerve stimulation, which is considered first-line therapy treatment for fecal incontinence, has shown good outcomes in the ileal pouch-anal anastomosis population and can improve symptoms in two-third of patients when offered [46].

Patients can also develop obstruction secondary to adhesive disease after surgery for stricture of the ileal pouch-anal anastomosis. Small bowel obstruction occurs in up to 40% of patients. This can occur secondary to adhesive disease or afferent limb syndrome, where an acute angulation occurs in the limb of the J-pouch [45]. Obstruction can also occur due to outlet obstruction secondary to stricture formation. Anal stricture occurs in approximately 13.6% of patients within 5 years, but that number can increase to 56% after 30 years [45, 47]. Stricture formation is also 8 times more likely after three-stage procedures compared to two-stage procedures with no differences in anastomotic leak or pelvic sepsis [48].

While ileal pouch-anal anastomosis minimizes the chance of developing colorectal cancer, there is still a small remnant rectal cuff as opposed to end ileostomy, where a remnant cuff is not necessary to form an anastomosis. Due to this remnant rectal cuff and anal transition zone, there is a small risk of dysplasia as a small amount of rectal mucosa remains when a stapled approach is used. A systematic review observed dysplasia in the mucosal remnant in 0–4.4% of patients after 10 or more years [30].

Pouch patients may also develop fistulas to their pouch. These fistulas can occur in the vagina, bladder, small bowel, or perianal skin. While not common, these can occur in 4% of patients. Primary treatment includes drainage of any associated abscess with draining seton placement. After adequate drainage, subsequent treatment options include advancement flaps, transvaginal repair, or mesenchymal stem cells. However, one third of patients who develop a fistula to their pouch do ultimately require pouch excision [47, 49–53].

Pouch failure can occur in up to 17% of J-pouch patients. While a subjective measure, chronic pouch failure is defined by patient factors such as stool frequency, urgency, incontinence, or chronic antibiotic-refractory pouchitis. Etiologies of pouch failure include mechanical outlet obstruction, pouch intussusception, efferent loop kinking, or emptying problems. While revision and reconstruction of the pouch is an option, many of these patients undergo either proximal diversion with a loop ileostomy or complete excision of the pouch with conversion to an end ileostomy [54].

Another important long-term outcome to consider after surgery is sexual function. Prior to surgery, approximately one-third of patients report reduced or absent sexual activity due to the severity of their ulcerative colitis. After ileal pouch-anal anastomosis, 25% report improvement in their sex life, while 16% report mild restrictions to their desired sexual activity. When separated by sex, 3% of men reported sexual dysfunction while 11% of women reported similar dysfunction [55]. The differences in sexual function between men and women also dissipate 1 year after surgery [56]. Female fertility can also be affected by both ulcerative colitis and total proctocolectomy. With chronic ulcerative colitis alone, female patients experience a medical fertility rate of 14.6%, which increases to 48% after open total proctocolectomy with ileal pouch-anal anastomosis [57]. The etiology is believed to be scarring and adhesive disease to the Fallopian tubes after pelvic dissection. After the introduction of laparoscopic surgery, female infertility rates have improved to 27% [58]. In terms of pregnancy after ileal pouch-anal anastomosis, women have no significant difference in pregnancy complications, labor, delivery complications, unplanned Cesarean section, or birth weight. Completion of successful gestation, pregnancy, and delivery also have no difference in functional outcomes of the pouch [59].

Patients also have financial considerations when choosing an operation. Due to the cost of biologic therapy, direct medical costs are lower after surgery when compared to before surgery. However, the two-year costs between medically managed and surgically managed patients are comparable. End ileostomy is approximately $8000

	End ileostomy	Ileal pouch anal anastomosis
Short-term outcomes		
Morbidity	=	=
Length of stay	=	=
Anastomotic leak		↑
Long-term outcomes		
Patient satisfaction	=	=
Fecal urgency		10%
Fecal incontinence		10%
Pouchitis		30–50%
Small bowel obstruction	=	=
Pouch fistula		4%
Pouch failure		17%
Finances		
Well-functioning pouch		↓
Pouchitis	↓	

Table 1.
Outcomes comparison between end ileostomy and ileal pouch anal anastomosis.

more expensive for patients than ileal pouch-anal anastomosis due to the cost of stoma supplies over a two-year period. In pouch patients who developed pouchitis, their two-year cost was $12,000 more expensive than end ileostomy patients [60]. When differentiating risk factors for medical financial toxicity, disease extent is more associated with increased cost compared to disease severity [61].

A summary comparing the short- and long-term outcomes after end ileostomy versus ileal pouch anal anastomosis is presented in **Table 1**.

6. Conclusion

With the advances in medical management, surgery for ulcerative colitis is becoming increasingly less common. Defining surgical indications such as failure of medical management becomes increasingly complex and involves multidisciplinary evaluation, collaboration, and decision-making. Once a consensus recommendation has been reached to proceed with surgery, patient factors such as comorbidities, severity of ulcerative colitis, steroid use, frailty, and fecal incontinence should be factored into surgical selection. Surgical options include total abdominal colectomy with end ileostomy, total proctocolectomy with end ileostomy, or total proctocolectomy with ileal pouch-anal anastomosis reconstruction in a three-, two-, or single-staged fashion. Knowledge of short-term outcomes, long-term outcomes, risks of malignancy, and pouch function is integral to conducting a true patient-centered selection of the operative approach. With appropriate preoperative and postoperative counseling, patient satisfaction is equal for a permanent end ileostomy and for restoration of intestinal continuity with an ileal pouch-anal anastomosis.

Conflict of interest

The authors declare no conflict of interest.

Author details

Jonathan Hughes[1], Sarai Krewson[2], Griffin Bryant[2] and Bethany Malone[1*]

1 Texas Health Fort Worth, Department of Surgery, Fort Worth, TX, USA

2 Burnett School of Medicine, Texas Christian University, Fort Worth, TX, USA

*Address all correspondence to: bcbmalone@gmail.com

References

[1] Le Berre C, Honap S, Peyrin-Biroulet L. Ulcerative colitis. The Lancet. 2023;**402**(10401):571-584

[2] Lightner AL, Pemberton JH, Dozois EJ, et al. The surgical management of inflammatory bowel disease. Current Problems in Surgery. 2017;**54**:172-250

[3] Samuel S, Ingle SB, Dhillon S, et al. Cumulative incidence and risk factors for hospitalization and surgery in a population-based cohort of ulcerative colitis. Inflammatory Bowel Diseases. 2013;**19**(9):1858-1866

[4] Rubin DT, Ananthakrishnan AN, Siegel CA, et al. ACG clinical guideline: Ulcerative colitis in adults. The American Journal of Gastroenterology. 2019;**114**:384-413

[5] Sethi K, Sethi-Arora K, Limdi JK. Health maintenance strategies in adults with inflammatory bowel disease. Clinics in Integrated Care. 2024;**23**:100191

[6] Narula N, Fine M, Colonbel JF, et al. Systematic review: Sequential rescue therapy in severe ulcerative colitis: Do the benefits outweigh the risks? Inflammatory Bowel Diseases. 2015;**21**:1683-1694

[7] Schäcke H, Döcke WD, Asadullah K. Mechanisms involved in the side effects of glucocorticoids. Pharmacology and Therapeutics. 2002;**96**:23-43

[8] Rutgeerts P, Löfberg R, Malchow H, et al. A comparison of budesonide with prednisolone for active Crohn's disease. New England Journal of Medicine. 1994;**331**:842-845

[9] Dignass A, Eliakim R, Magro F, et al. Second European evidence-based consensus on the diagnosis and management of ulcerative colitis part 1: Definitions and diagnosis. Journal of Crohn's and Colitis. 2012;**6**:965-990

[10] Munkholm P, Langholz E, Davidsen M, et al. Frequency of glucocorticoid resistance and dependency in Crohn's disease. Gut. 1994;**35**:360-362

[11] Faubion WA, Loftus EV, Harmsen WS, et al. The natural history of corticosteroid therapy for inflammatory bowel disease: A population-based study. Gastroenterology. 2001;**121**:255-260

[12] Filipe V, Allen PB, Peyrin-Biroulet L. Self-medication with steroids in inflammatory bowel disease. Digestive and Liver Disease. 2016;**48**(1):23-26

[13] DeLeon M, Stocchi L. Elective and emergent surgery in the ulcerative colitis patient. Clinics in Colon and Rectal Surgery. 2022;**35**(6):437-444

[14] Eaden J, Abrams K, Mayberry J. The risk of colorectal cancer in ulcerative colitis: A meta-analysis. Gut. 2001;**48**(4):526-535

[15] Munie S, Hyman N, Osler T. Fate of the rectal stump after subtotal colectomy for ulcerative colitis in the era of ileal pouch-anal anastomosis. JAMA Surgery. 2013;**148**(5):408-411

[16] Malone B. J-pouch configuration of ileal pouch anal anastomosis. 2025. Ink on paper

[17] Lovegrove RE, Heriot AG, Constantinides V, et al. Meta-analysis of short-term and long-term outcomes of J, W, and S ileal reservoirs for restorative proctocolectomy. Colorectal Disease. 2006;**9**(4):310-320

[18] McCormick PH, Guest GD, Clark AJ, et al. The ideal ileal-pouch design: A long-term randomized control trial of J- vs W-pouch construction. Diseases of the Colon and Rectum. 2012;**55**(12):1251-1257

[19] Mukewar S, Wu X, Lopez R, et al. Comparison of long-term outcomes of S and J pouches and continent ileostomies in ulcerative colitis patients with restorative proctocolectomy – Experience in subspecialty pouch center. Journal of Crohn's and Colitis. 2014;**8**(10):1227-1236

[20] Weston-Petrides GK, Lovegrove RE, Tilney HS. Comparison of outcomes after restorative proctocolectomy with or without defunctioning ileostomy. Archives of Surgery. 2008;**143**(4):406-412

[21] Kirat HT, Remzi FH. Technical aspects of ileoanal pouch surgery in patients with ulcerative colitis. Clinics in Colon and Rectal Surgery. 2010;**23**(4):239-247

[22] Balachandran R, TØttrup A. Safety of proctocolectomy for ulcerative colitis under elective and non-elective circumstances: Preoperative corticosteroid treatment worsens outcome. Digestive Surgery. 2015;**32**(4):251-257

[23] Braga M, Vignali A, Gianotti L, et al. Laparoscopic versus open colorectal surgery. Annals of Surgery. 2002;**236**(6):759-767

[24] Hernandas AK, Jenkins JT. Laparoscopic pouch surgery in ulcerative colitis. Annals of Gastroenterology. 2012;**25**(4):309-316

[25] Tan JJY, Tjandra JJ. Laparoscopic surgery for ulcerative colitis – A meta analysis. Colorectal Disease. 2006;**8**(8):626-636

[26] Warps ALK, Zwanenburg ES, Dekker JWT, et al. Laparoscopic versus open colorectal surgery in the emergency setting. Annals of Surgery Open. 2021;**2**(3):e097

[27] Panteleimonitis S, Al-Dhaheri M, Parvaiz A, et al. Short-term outcomes in robotic vs laparoscopic ileal pouch-anal anastomosis surgery: A propensity score match study. Langenbeck's Archives of Surgery. 2023;**408**:175

[28] Gebhardt JM, Werner N, Stroux A, et al. Robotic-assisted versus laparoscopic proctectomy with ileal pouch-anal anastomosis for ulcerative colitis: An analysis of clinical and financial outcomes from a tertiary referral center. Journal of Clinical Medicine. 2022;**11**(21):6561

[29] Zaman S, Mohamedahmed AYY, Abdelrahman W, et al. Minimally invasive surgery for inflammatory bowel disease: A systematic review and meta-analysis of robotic versus laparoscopic surgical techniques. Journal of Crohn's and Colitis. 2024;**18**(8):1342-1355

[30] Scoglio D, Ali UA, Fichera A. Surgical treatment of ulcerative colitis: Ileorectal vs ileal pouch-anal anastomosis. World Journal of Gastroenterology. 2014;**20**(37):13211-13218

[31] Lissel M, Omidy S, et al. The handling of the rectal stump does not affect severe morbidity after subtotal colectomy for ulcerative colitis: A retrospective cohort study. Scandinavian Journal of Surgery. 2020;**109**(3):238-243

[32] Lee GC, Bhama AR. Minimally invasive and robotic surgery for ulcerative colitis. Clinics in Colon and Rectal Surgery. 2022;**35**(6):463-468

[33] Heuthorst L, Wasmann KA, Reijntjes MA, Hompes R, Buskens CJ,

Bemelman WA, et al. Ileal pouch-anal anastomosis complications and pouch failure: A systematic review and meta-analysis. Annals of Surgery Open. 2021;**2**(2):e074

[34] Chung TP, Fleshman J, Birnbaum E, et al. Laparoscopic vs open total abdominal colectomy for severe colitis impact on recovery and subsequent completion restorative proctectomy. Diseases of the Colon & Rectum. 2009;**52**(1):4-10

[35] Kim JC, Lee JL, Yoon YS, et al. Entirely robot-assisted total colectomy/ total proctocolectomy compared with a laparoscopic approach. Surgical Laparoscopy, Endoscopy, and Percutaneous Techniques. 2021;**31**(4):428-433

[36] Bergamaschi R, Pessaux P, Arnaud JP. Comparison of conventional and laparoscopic ileocolic resection for Crohn's disease. Diseases of the Colon and Rectum. 2003;**46**(8):1129-1133

[37] Murphy PB, Khot Z, Vogt KN, et al. Quality of life after total proctocolectomy with ileostomy of IPAA: A systematic review. Diseases of the Colon and Rectum. 2015;**58**:899-908

[38] Heuschen UA, Autschbach F, et al. Long-term follow-up after ileoanal pouch procedure. Diseases of the Colon and Rectum. 2001;**44**:487-499

[39] Barnes EL, Boynton MH, DeWalt DA, et al. Patient reported outcome assessments used in the evaluation of patients after ileal pouch-anal anastomosis: A systematic review. Gastro Hep Advances. 2023;**2**(8):1044-1049

[40] Selvaggi F, Giuliani A, Gallo C, Signoriello G, Riegler G, Canonico S. Randomized, controlled trial to compare the J-pouch and W-pouch configurations for ulcerative colitis in the maturation period. Diseases of the Colon and Rectum. 2000;**43**(5):615-620

[41] Khera AJ, Chase JW, Salzberg M, et al. Determinants of long-term function and general well-being in patients with an ileoanal pouch. JGH Open. 2021;**5**(1):91-98

[42] van Overstraeten d B, Wolthuis AM, Verneire S, et al. Long-term functional outcome after ileal pouch anal anastomosis in 191 patients with ulcerative colitis. Journal of Crohn's and Colitis. 2014;**8**(10):1261-1266

[43] Lee GC, Cavallaro PM, Savitt LR, et al. Bowel function after j-pouch may be more complex than previously appreciated: A comprehensive analysis to highlight existing knowledge gaps. Diseases of the Colon and Rectum. 2020;**63**:207-216

[44] Hahnloser D, Pemberton JH, Wolff BG, Larson DR, Crownhart BS, Dozois RR. Results at up to 20 years after ileal pouch-anal anastomosis for chronic ulcerative colitis. The British Journal of Surgery. 2007;**94**(3):333-340

[45] Lee GC, Deery SE, Kunitake H, et al. Comparable perioperative outcomes, long-term outcomes, and quality of life in a retrospective analysis of ulcerative colitis patients following 2-stage versus 3-stage proctocolectomy with ileal pouch-anal anastomosis. International Journal of Colorectal Disease. 2019;**34**(3):491-499

[46] Seifarth C, Slavova N, Degro C, et al. Sacral nerve stimulation in patients with ileal pouch-anal anastomosis. International Journal of Colorectal Disease. 2021;**36**(9):1937-1943

[47] Fazio VW, Kiran RP, Remzi FH, et al. Ileal pouch anal anastomosis:

Analysis of outcome and quality of life in 3707 patients. Annals of Surgery. 2013;**257**(4):679-685

[48] Hicks CW, Hodin RA, Bordeianou L. Possible overuse of 3-stage procedures for active ulcerative colitis. JAMA Surgery. 2013;**148**(7):658-664

[49] Mallick IH, Hull TL, Remzi FH, Kiran RP. Management and outcome of pouch-vaginal fistulas after IPAA surgery. Diseases of the Colon and Rectum. 2014;**57**(4):490-496

[50] Sagar RC, Thornton M, Herd A, Brayshaw I, Sagar PM. Transvaginal repair of recurrent pouch-vaginal fistula. Colorectal Disease. 2014;**16**(12):O440-O442

[51] Garcia-Olmo D, Herreros D, Pascual I, et al. Expanded adipose-derived stem cells for the treatment of complex perianal fistula: A phase II clinical trial. Diseases of the Colon and Rectum. 2009;**52**(1):79-86

[52] Ciccocioppo R, Bernardo ME, Sgarella A, et al. Autologous bone marrow-derived mesenchymal stromal cells in the treatment of fistulising Crohn's disease. Gut. 2011;**60**(6):788-798

[53] de la Portilla F, Alba F, Garcia-Olmo D, Herrerias JM, Gonzalez FX, Galindo A. Expanded allogeneic adipose-derived stem cells (eASCs) for the treatment of complex perianal fistula in Crohn's disease: Results from a multicenter phase I/IIa clinical trial. International Journal of Colorectal Disease. 2013;**28**(3):313-323

[54] Reijntjes MA, Bocharewicz EK, Hompes R, et al. Incidence and causes of failure in various anatomical pouch designs 20 years after surgical primary ileal-pouch anal anastomosis construction. International Journal of Colorectal Diseases. 2022;**37**(12):2491-2499

[55] Farouk R, Pemberton JH, Wolff BG, et al. Functional outcomes after ileal pouch-anal anastomosis for chronic ulcerative colitis. Annals of Surgery. 2000;**231**(6):919-926

[56] Davies RJ, O'Connor BI, Victor C, MacRae HM, Cohen Z, McLeod RS. A prospective evaluation of sexual function and quality of life after ileal pouch-anal anastomosis. Diseases of the Colon and Rectum. 2008;**51**(7):1032-1035

[57] Waljee A, Waljee J, Morris AM, Higgins PD. Threefold increased risk of infertility: A meta-analysis of infertility after ileal pouch anal anastomosis in ulcerative colitis. Gut. 2006;**55**(11):1575-1580

[58] Beyer-Berjot L, Maggiori L, Birnbaum D, Lefevre JH, Berdah S, Panis Y. A total laparoscopic approach reduces the infertility rate after ileal pouch-anal anastomosis: A 2-center study. Annals of Surgery. 2013;**258**(2):275-282

[59] Hahnloser D, Pemberton JH, Wolff BG, et al. Pregnancy and delivery before and after ileal pouch-anal anastomosis for inflammatory bowel disease: Immediate and long-term consequences and outcomes. Diseases of the Colon and Rectum. 2004;**47**(7):1127-1135

[60] Holubar SD, Pendlimari R, Loftus EV, et al. Drivers of cost after surgical and medical therapy for chronic ulcerative colitis: A nested case-cohort study in Olmsted County, Minnesota. Diseases of the Colon & Rectum. 2012;**55**:1258-1265

[61] Kappelman MD, Rifas-Shiman SL, Porter CQ, et al. Direct health care costs of Crohn's disease and ulcerative colitis in US children and adults. Gastroenterology. 2008;**135**:1907-1913

Chapter 6

Evidence-Based Complementary Therapies for the Management of Ulcerative Colitis

Vijay Kondreddy, Bhavani Gadiraju and Jhansi Magisetty

Abstract

Ulcerative colitis (UC), a chronic inflammatory bowel disease, profoundly affects patients' quality of life through persistent gastrointestinal symptoms and systemic complications. Conventional therapies include aminosalicylates, corticosteroids, immunomodulators, and biologics, yet many patients experience limited effectiveness and severe adverse effects. This limitation has spurred a rising interest in complementary therapies, offering promising avenues for symptom management and enhancement of overall well-being. This chapter explores an array of complementary approaches, such as dietary modifications, herbal supplements, prebiotics, and probiotics. By focusing on the robust empirical evidence, mechanisms of action, and practical implementation of these therapies.

Keywords: ulcerative colitis, complementary therapies, dietary and herbal interventions, immunomodulators, cytokines

1. Introduction

Ulcerative colitis and Crohn's disease, collectively known as inflammatory bowel disease (IBD), are chronic conditions associated with significant morbidity and mortality [1, 2]. Ulcerative colitis (UC) is a chronic inflammatory bowel disease marked by immune-related inflammation and the development of ulcers on the intestinal mucosal surface [3, 4]. The precise cause of UC is not well understood [5]. Common symptoms include chronic diarrhea, bloody stools, and abdominal discomfort [6]. Both the incidence and prevalence of UC have been increasing worldwide [7]. Despite major advances in our understanding of intestinal inflammation over the past two decades, driven by experimental animal models, the exact causes of these diseases remain unknown [8]. Current treatments for UC, such as corticosteroids and immunosuppressants, often prove insufficient and come with considerable adverse effects [9]. While these conventional therapies can manage symptoms and induce remission, they do not provide a cure and may not work for all patients. Moreover, the significant side effects associated with these treatments can further complicate patient care, underscoring the need for safer and more effective therapeutic options

 IntechOpen

[10, 11]. Aminosalicylic acids (ASAs), particularly mesalamine (5-ASA) administered orally or via enema, are the primary treatments for UC [12]. However, patients who do not respond to 5-ASA often turn to corticosteroids or immunomodulators to manage the condition, despite the potential for adverse effects. This has led to a growing demand for new compounds capable of inducing and maintaining remission in UC without significant side effects [13]. This chapter explores emerging therapeutic strategies that hold promise for the future treatment of ulcerative colitis. These novel approaches aim to address the limitations of existing treatments by offering improved efficacy and a better safety profile. The focus is on various innovative therapies, including dietary modifications, herbal supplements, prebiotics, probiotics, and other complementary approaches. By examining the latest research findings and clinical experiences, this chapter highlights the potential of these emerging therapies to improve patient outcomes and quality of life.

2. Complementary therapies for ulcerative colitis (UC)

Patients with inflammatory bowel disease (IBD) often experience symptoms such as abdominal discomfort, diarrhea, the presence of blood in their stools, and mucosal damage [14]. A prompt and precise diagnosis, an assessment of the patient's risk of unfavorable outcomes, and the onset of efficient, secure, and acceptable medical therapies are all essential components of UC management. A prolonged and durable period of steroid-free remission, accompanied by suitable psychosocial support, a normal health-related quality of life (QoL), the avoidance of morbidity, including hospitalization and surgery, and the prevention of cancer, represent the ideal course of treatment. Mucosal healing is a new objective in the therapy of ulcerative colitis [15]. Knowing the best preventive, therapeutic, and diagnostic techniques is essential to achieving these objectives.

2.1 Prebiotics

Prebiotics are non-digestible fiber compounds that promote the growth of beneficial bacteria in the gut, such as bifidobacteria and lactobacilli [16]. Prebiotics help maintain a balanced gut microbiome, support digestive health, and enhance immune function [17]. The most common types of prebiotics include fructo-oligosaccharides (FOS), inulin, galacto-oligosaccharides (GOS), and resistant starches [18]. Inulin, found in chicory root, ferments in the colon to produce short-chain fatty acids (SCFAs) like butyrate, which has anti-inflammatory properties [19]. By modulating the gut microbiota and enhancing the immune response, prebiotics play a crucial role in managing colitis and promoting overall gut health. Koleva et al. demonstrated that fructo-oligosaccharides (FOS) and inulin reduce Clostridium cluster XI and promote Bifidobacterium spp. in rats, leading to decreased intestinal inflammation [20]. Hoentjen et al. found that a prebiotic combination of inulin-type fructans reduced colitis in HLA-B27 transgenic rats, linked to gut microbiota changes, and increased TGF-β [21]. Wang et al. showed that stachyose improved weight recovery, reduced colonic damage, and corrected microbiota imbalances in UC mice [22]. Lunken et al. reported that inulin-type fructans-enriched enteral nutrition (ENN) reduced colitis severity in a T-cell transfer model, promoting beneficial microbes

Author	Year	Type of study	Study design	Primary outcome	Results
Hoentjen et al.	2005	Animal model (HLA-B27 rats)	Prebiotic treatment	Reduction of colitis, microbiota changes, immunomodulation	Reduced colitis, increased bifidobacteria, and TGF-β levels
Casellas et al.	2007	Clinical study	Oligofructose-enriched inulin	Intestinal inflammation reduction	Lowered fecal calprotectin levels
Vulevic et al.	2008	Clinical study	GOS treatment	Impact on beneficial bacteria, immune response	Increased bifidobacteria and lactobacilli, reduced harmful bacteria, enhanced immune response
Koleva et al.	2012	Animal model (Rats)	Prebiotic (FOS) treatment	Impact on gut microbiota and intestinal inflammation	Promoted Bifidobacterium spp., reduced Clostridium, decreased inflammation
Lunken et al.	2021	Animal model (T-cell transfer mice)	EEN with inulin	Effects on mucus, T-cell subsets, and microbiota	Improved mucus integrity, expanded anti-inflammatory T-cell subsets, increased beneficial microbes
Li et al.	2021	Clinical study	XOS treatment	Impact on microflora and inflammation	Increased bifidobacteria, reduced harmful bacteria, improved inflammation
Wang et al.	2023	Animal model (C57BL/6 mice)	Prebiotic (Stachyose)	Recovery of body weight, tissue damage reduction, microbiota restoration	Improved weight recovery, reduced inflammation, restored microbiota balance

Table 1.
Summary of evidence on the effects of prebiotic supplementation in UC patients.

and anti-inflammatory T-cells [23]. Vulevic et al. demonstrated that galactooligosaccharides (GOS) promoted beneficial bacteria and enhanced immune response [24]. Casellas et al. found that oligofructose-enriched inulin reduced intestinal inflammation in UC patients, as evidenced by lower fecal calprotectin levels [25]. Suzuki et al. showed that the bifidogenic growth stimulator (BGS) improved microflora balance, enhancing colonic health and preventing damage [26]. Li et al. demonstrated that xylo-oligosaccharide (XOS) promoted bifidobacteria, reducing harmful bacteria and alleviating UC symptoms [27]. Prebiotics can help modulate intestinal flora, reducing UC's severity (**Table 1**).

2.2 Probiotics

Probiotics are live microorganisms that confer health benefits to the host when administered in adequate amounts. They are often used to improve gut health by restoring the natural balance of gut flora, which can be disrupted in conditions like ulcerative colitis (UC) [28]. Many studies have shown that intestinal microflora plays a major role in the pathogenesis of ulcerative colitis [29]. Probiotics are among the most popular CAM therapies and come in various forms, including single or multiple strains of bacteria and/or yeast [30]. Probiotics are hypothesized to have anti-inflammatory properties and to influence immune-modulatory pathways, including phosphoinositide 3-kinase/Akt pathway inhibition and nuclear factor κ–light chain enhancer of activated B cells (NF-κB) pathway inhibition [31–33]. They may also affect the expression of Toll-like receptors and inflammatory cytokines. Several clinical studies have investigated the efficacy of probiotics in managing UC. A meta-analysis by Sartor of randomized controlled trials found that probiotics, particularly formulations containing multiple strains of beneficial bacteria, can induce remission and maintain disease stability in UC patients [34]. In patients with mild-to-moderate ulcerative colitis (UC), the probiotic formulation VSL#3 has been shown to induce remission. A study conducted by Tursi et al. demonstrated that VSL#3 led to a nearly 50% reduction in the disease activity index compared to placebo [35]. Studies conducted by Miele et al. and Bibiloni et al. have shown that when VSL#3 is administered alongside standard therapies, it significantly enhances clinical remission and reduces endoscopic severity in patients with ulcerative colitis [36, 37]. A study by Kruis et al. found that the probiotic strain *Escherichia coli* Nissle 1917 is as effective as mesalamine in regulating remission in patients with ulcerative colitis [29]. The studies demonstrated that probiotics could reduce the frequency and severity of flare-ups, improve symptoms such as abdominal pain and diarrhea, and promote mucosal healing [15]. The exact mechanisms by which probiotics exert their effects may include modulating the immune response, enhancing gut barrier function, and reducing pathogenic bacterial colonization (**Table 2**) [38, 39].

Author	Year	Type of study	Study design	Primary outcome	Results
Sartor et al.	2004	Meta-analysis (RCTs)	Multiple RCTs on probiotics in UC	Effectiveness of probiotics in inducing/ remission in UC	Probiotics, especially multi-strain formulations, can induce remission and maintain disease stability in UC
Tursi et al.	2010	Randomized controlled trial (RCT)	VSL#3 (3600 billion CFU/day) vs. placebo for 8 weeks in relapsing UC patients	Reduction in UC Disease Activity Index (UCDAI), remission, and improvement in rectal bleeding	VSL#3 reduced the disease activity index by nearly 50% compared to placebo
Bibiloni et al. and Miele et al.	2005 and 2009	Randomized controlled trial (RCT)	VSL#3 with standard therapies in UC	Clinical remission and endoscopic severity	VSL#3 improved clinical remission and reduced endoscopic severity when combined with standard therapies
Kruis et al.	2004	Randomized controlled trial (RCT)	*E. coli* Nissle 1917 vs. mesalamine	Remission maintenance	*E. coli* Nissle 1917 is as effective as mesalamine in maintaining remission

Table 2.
Summary of evidence on the effects of probiotic supplementation in UC patients.

2.3 Curcumin

Curcumin is the primary bioactive compound found in turmeric (*Curcuma longa*). It has strong anti-inflammatory, antioxidant, and anti-cancer properties [40]. In the context of ulcerative colitis (UC), curcumin is believed to help reduce inflammation and support mucosal healing [41]. It has been shown to have anti-inflammatory and antioxidant properties on human lymphocytes and gut epithelial cell lines and reduces histologic features of inflammation and colitis in mice [42, 43]. A randomized, double-blind, placebo-controlled trial conducted by Hanai et al. over 6 months demonstrated that curcumin, in combination with standard mesalamine treatment, significantly improved clinical and endoscopic remission rates in patients with mild-to-moderate UC [42]. In a study conducted by Sugimoto et al. on TNBS-induced colitis in mice, it was found that administering curcumin resulted in a significant reduction in body weight loss compared to the placebo group [41]. Another study conducted by Ukil et al. revealed that curcumin-pretreated mice with TNBS-induced colitis there is a preferential expression of Th1 and Th2 cytokines in the mucosa of the colon. There has been a repression in the NF-kB activation [44]. Jagetia and Aggarwal demonstrated that curcumin is capable of mitigating the expression of several pro-inflammatory cytokines such as TNF, ILs, and chemokines by modulating the expression of transcription factor NF-kB [45]. Patients receiving curcumin had a relapse rate of 4.7%, compared to 20.5% in the placebo group, indicating its potential as an effective adjunct therapy in UC management (**Table 3**) [46].

Author	Year	Type of study	Study design	Primary outcome	Results
Sugimoto et al.	2002	Animal study	TNBS-induced colitis in mice; curcumin vs. placebo	Body weight loss reduction in colitis mode	Curcumin led to significantly less weight loss compared to the placebo group
Ukil et al.	2003	Animal study	TNBS-induced colitis in mice; curcumin-pretreated	Cytokine expression (Th1, Th2), NF-kB activity	Repression of NF-kB activation and cytokine modulation in curcumin-treated mice
Hanai et al.	2006	RCT	6-month trial; curcumin + mesalamine vs. placebo	Clinical and endoscopic remission	Significant improvement in remission rates; relapse rate 4.7% for the curcumin group vs. 20.5% for the placebo
Jagetia et al.	2007	In vitro	Evaluation of cytokine modulation by curcumin	Pro-inflammatory cytokines (TNF, ILs) expression	Curcumin mitigated pro-inflammatory cytokines by modulating NF-kB activity

Table 3.
Summary of evidence on effects of curcumin supplementation in UC patients.

2.4 Fish oil

Fish oil is a rich source of omega-3 fatty acids (n-3 PUFAs), particularly eicosapentaenoic acid (EPA) and docosahexaenoic acid (DHA) [47–49]. EPA and DHA modulate the expression of several transcription factors that include hepatic nuclear factor (HNF)-4α, liver X receptors (LXRs), and peroxisome proliferator-activated receptors (PPARs) which have a critical role in IBD [50]. Activation of PPARs by n-3 PUFAs inhibits the NF-kB signaling pathway, thereby reducing the transcription of NF-kB-dependent genes such as COX-2, IL-6, TNF-α, and other chemokines implicated in IBD [51]. The clinical efficacy of fish oil in UC has been investigated in several studies. In a study conducted by Magisetty et al., rats with DSS-induced colitis pretreated with n-3 PUFAs showed dysregulation of colitis-associated genes including Etv3, clec4d, CD180, CD72, Megf11, and Angptl4 [52]. A study conducted by Reddy et al. demonstrated that n-3 polyunsaturated fatty acids (PUFAs) significantly improved body weight loss, rectal bleeding, and mortality rate in DSS-induced colitis rats. This improvement was attributed to the downregulation of myeloperoxidase activity, nitric oxide, prostaglandin E2, TNF-α, IL-6, IL-8, COX-2, and iNOS levels [53]. McLean et al. conducted a double-blind, placebo-controlled trial and found that fish oil supplementation led to a significant reduction in rectal bleeding and stool frequency, two key symptoms of UC [54]. An RCT done by Seidner et al. found that EPA (1 g twice daily) was associated with significant reductions in fecal calprotectin levels and maintenance of remission compared to placebo [55]. The variability in outcomes may be due to differences in dosages and the ratios of EPA to DHA used in these studies (**Table 4**).

Author	Year	Type of study	Study design	Primary outcome	Results
McLean et al.	2005	Double-blind, placebo RCT	Fish oil supplementation vs. placebo	Rectal bleeding, stool frequency	Fish oil significantly reduced rectal bleeding and stool frequency
Siedner et al.	2005	Randomized controlled trial	EPA (1 g twice daily) vs. placebo	Fecal calprotectin, remission maintenance	EPA led to significant reductions in fecal calprotectin and improved remission maintenance
Vijay et al.	2016	Animal study	DSS-induced colitis; n-3 PUFA supplementation	Inflammatory markers, rectal bleeding, mortality	n-3 PUFAs significantly reduced rectal bleeding, body weight loss, and inflammation
Jhansi et al.	2024	Animal study	DSS-induced colitis; n-3 PUFA supplementation	Colitis-associated gene dysregulation (Etv3, Angptl4)	n-3 PUFAs showed dysregulation of genes related to colitis, including Etv3, CD72, and Angptl4

Table 4.
Summary of evidence on the effects of curcumin supplementation in UC patients.

2.5 Herbal medicines

2.5.1 Andrographis paniculata

Andrographis paniculata (AP), a member of the plant family Acanthaceae, is an herbal remedy used in China and many other Asian countries [56]. It is commonly known as "King of Bitters." It is known for its anti-inflammatory, antiviral, and immune-boosting properties [57]. In a study by Gao et al., andrographolide, the most active phytochemical in *Andrographis paniculata* (AP) and its derivative CX-10, significantly reduced body weight loss, colon length shortening, and disease activity index (DAI) in mice with DSS-induced colitis [58, 59]. In a study conducted by Sandborn et al., a multicenter RCT of patients with active mild-to-moderate UC, its extract, HMPL-004, produced similar rates of clinical remission, response, and endoscopic remission when compared with 5-ASAs at 8 weeks. The study found that the extract was as effective as mesalamine in reducing disease activity and improving quality of life, suggesting it could be a viable alternative or adjunct to conventional treatments [60]. In another study by Michelsen et al., HMPL-004 treatment in mice with MC-induced colitis downregulated the expression of TNF-α, IL-1β, IFN-γ, and IL-22 [61]. Hence, AP can be used as an alternative for inducing remission and mitigating the disease symptoms in UC patients.

2.5.2 *Indigo Naturalis*

Indigo Naturalis (IN), also known as Qing Dai, is a traditional Chinese herbal medicine extracted from Indigofera Tinctora and is known for its anti-inflammatory and immunomodulatory effects [62, 63]. The anti-inflammatory effect of IN is thought to be due to inhibition of TNF-α, interleukin (IL)-1 and -6, and NF-κB, as well as promotion of IL-22 production [64]. Clinical studies have shown promising results with Indigo Naturalis in the attenuation of UC. A study by Yokote et al. demonstrated that treatment with Indigo Naturalis confers resistance to ferroptosis in cells, thereby protecting the intestinal epithelium [65]. Kawai et al. demonstrated that Indigo Naturalis ameliorated murine colitis through the activation of AhR signaling [66]. Li et al. demonstrated that Indirubin, a component of Indigo Naturalis, significantly mitigated DSS-induced weight loss in UC mice, improved colon length, and altered the expression of various pro-inflammatory factors, including TNF-α, IL-6, IFN-γ, COX-2, iNOS, and MPO activity [67]. In an RCT conducted by Naganuma et al. Indigo Naturalis increased the expression of proteins and cytokines related to colonic mucosal repair while decreasing myeloperoxidase activity and inflammatory cytokine expression in rat models of colitis induced by dextran sodium sulfate [68]. A small, open-label pilot study by Wang et al. found that patients treated with Indigo Naturalis experienced significant improvements in clinical symptoms and endoscopic scores (**Table 5**) [69].

Author	Year	Type of study	Study design	Primary outcome	Results
Andrographis paniculata					
Sandborn et al.	2013	Randomized controlled trial	Multicenter RCT; HMPL-004 vs. 5-ASA	Clinical remission, endoscopic remission	HMPL-004 showed similar efficacy to mesalamine in reducing disease activity in patients with UC
Michelsen et al.	2013	Animal study	MC-induced colitis in mice; HMPL-004 treatment	Inflammatory cytokine expression	HMPL-004 downregulated pro-inflammatory cytokines TNF-α, IL-1β, IFN-γ, and IL-22

Author	Year	Type of study	Study design	Primary outcome	Results
Gao et al.	2018	Animal study	DSS-induced colitis in mice; andrographolide treatment	Body weight, colon length, DAI	Andrographolide reduced body weight loss, colon length shortening, and DAI in colitis-induced mice
Indigo Naturalis					
Li et al.	2014	Animal study	DSS-induced colitis in mice; Indirubin component	Body weight, colon length, inflammatory markers	Mitigated weight loss, improved colon length, and reduced pro-inflammatory factors in UC mice
Wang et al.	2017	Open-label pilot study	UC patients; Indigo Naturalis treatment	Clinical symptoms, endoscopic scores	Clinical symptoms, endoscopic scores
Kawai et al.	2017	Animal study	Murine colitis model; Indigo Naturalis treatment	AhR signaling activation	Ameliorated murine colitis through activation of AhR signaling
Naganuma et al.	2018	Randomized controlled trial	DSS-induced colitis in rats; Indigo Naturalis vs. placebo	Mucosal repair, cytokine expression, MPO activity	Increased mucosal repair proteins, decreased MPO activity, and inflammatory cytokines
Yokote et al.	2023	In vitro study	Indigo Naturalis treatment	Ferroptosis resistance	Shielded the intestinal epithelial cells by conferring resistance to ferroptosis

Table 5.
Summary of evidence on the effects of herbal supplementation in UC patients.

2.6 Other botanical remedies

2.6.1 *Artemisia absinthium (worm wood)*

Artemisia absinthium, commonly known as wormwood, is an herb traditionally used in herbal medicine for its anti-inflammatory and antimicrobial properties [70]. Recent interest has focused on its potential benefits in managing ulcerative colitis (UC). Studies suggest that the bioactive compounds in wormwood, particularly artemisinin and its derivatives, may help reduce inflammation by modulating immune responses and inhibiting pro-inflammatory cytokines such as tumor necrosis factor-alpha (TNF-α) [71, 72]. These properties make *Artemisia absinthium* a promising adjunctive therapy in UC, potentially aiding in symptom reduction and improving the quality of life for patients. Two randomized controlled trials (RCTs) have provided promising insights into its efficacy [73, 74]. In the first trial, 20 patients with ulcerative colitis were assigned to receive standard treatment or standard treatment supplemented with *Artemisia absinthium* over 6 weeks. The group receiving wormwood showed a significant reduction in disease activity and associated symptoms, including a marked decrease in depressive symptoms and an improvement in overall quality of life, which was insignificant in the control groups. Moreover, a significant reduction in the levels of tumor necrosis factor-alpha (TNF-α), a pro-inflammatory cytokine, was observed in the wormwood group, indicating a potential anti-inflammatory effect [75]. The second study by Omer et al. focused on the effects of wormwood in conjunction with a tapering regimen of steroids or prednisolone in ulcerative colitis patients. This study followed 40 patients over 20 weeks, assessing outcomes such as symptom severity, quality of life, depression, and subjective well-being. The wormwood group experienced a significant reduction in symptoms at Weeks 6, 8, and 20, and reported improved well-being at Weeks 8, 10, and 12. These findings suggest that wormwood may help reduce dependence on steroid medications while improving patient well-being [74].

2.6.2 *Boswellia serrata*

Boswellia serrata, also known as Indian frankincense, is a resinous plant known for its potent anti-inflammatory properties, attributed to compounds called boswellic acids [76]. Boswellic acid, the major constituent of Boswellia, was shown to inhibit NF-kB signaling pathways in macrophages in a mouse model of psoriasis, markedly decreasing the production of the pro-inflammatory cytokines TNF-α, and the chemokine MCP-1 [77]. In addition, Stanke-Labesque et al. performed in vitro studies and animal models and demonstrated that boswellic acid inhibits 5-lipoxygenase selectively and has anti-inflammatory and anti-proliferative effects [78]. A study by Siemoneit et al. has shown that the action of boswellic acid is likely through mechanisms other than the inhibition of prostaglandin synthesis [79]. In a randomized controlled trial conducted by Gupta et al., *Boswellia serrata* extract demonstrated efficacy comparable to sulfasalazine, a standard treatment for UC, in maintaining remission. Patients receiving Boswellia experienced significant improvements in symptoms, suggesting it is a potential therapeutic option for UC [80].

2.6.3 *Aloe vera*

Aloe vera is a succulent plant known for its healing and anti-inflammatory properties. It is commonly used in treating various skin conditions and has also been explored for gastrointestinal disorders [81]. Langmead et al. conducted a randomized double-blind study involving patients with active UC and found that aloe vera gel significantly improved clinical response and remission rates compared to placebo. Nine (30%), eleven (37%), and fourteen (47%), respectively, of the thirty patients who received aloe vera experienced clinical remission, improvement, and response. In contrast, one (7%), one (7%), and two (14%; $P < 0.05$) of the fourteen patients who received a placebo experienced these comparable outcomes (using a 2:1 *A. vera*: placebo randomization schedule). During treatment with *A. vera*, but not with a placebo, there was a significant decrease in the Simple Clinical Colitis Activity Index and histological scores [82]. Another study by Bahrami et al. in acetic acid-induced UC rats pretreated with a 50 mg/kg dose of aloe vera showed reduced inflammation, ulcers, and tissue damage compared with the negative control [83]. The study highlighted aloe vera's potential as a complementary treatment, particularly for its soothing and anti-inflammatory effects on the gut mucosa.

2.6.4 *Germinated barley*

Germinated barley is a dietary supplement high in dietary fiber, which helps modulate gut flora and reduce inflammation. A clinical trial demonstrated that supplementation with germinated barley could reduce UC symptoms and promote mucosal healing [84, 85]. Patients in the study showed improvements in stool consistency and frequency, indicating its potential as a supportive therapy for UC [86]. The germinated barley, when given alongside the standard therapy for a group of UC patients, showed a significant decrease in the usage of corticosteroids after 3 months of this therapy, and after 12 months, the severity of clinical symptoms and the recurrence rate of UC in patients who achieved remission were significantly lower in the intervention group compared to the control group [87].

2.6.5 Wheatgrass juice (Triticum aestivum)

Wheatgrass juice is derived from the young shoots of the wheat plant. It is rich in chlorophyll, antioxidants, vitamins, and minerals and is believed to have detoxifying and anti-inflammatory properties [30]. A pilot study assessing the effects of wheatgrass juice in patients with active UC found that it reduced rectal bleeding, abdominal pain, and disease severity. The study suggested that wheatgrass juice might have a beneficial role in managing UC symptoms, although more extensive research is needed [88].

2.6.6 Chamomile

Chamomile is an herb known for its calming effects and anti-inflammatory properties. It is commonly used in herbal teas and traditional medicine [89]. With volatile acids, flavon glycosides, and hydroxycumarines as their primary constituents, the dry extract of chamomile flowers has anti-inflammatory, antibacterial, spasmolytic, and ulcer-protective properties [90]. Chamomile extract has been studied for its potential benefits in UC. A study by Menghini et al. in the LPS-induced acute colitis in rats pretreated with chamomile extract has shown a significant reduction in the production of MPO, IL-6, NF-kB, TNF-α, and PGE_2, which is as effective as sulfasalazine (**Table 6**) [91].

Author	Year	Type of study	Study design	Primary outcome	Results
Artemisia absinthium (worm wood)					
Omer et al.	2007	Clinical Trial (20 weeks)	Wormwood with tapering steroids in UC	Reduction in symptom severity at Weeks 6, 8, 20.	65% remission in the wormwood group (90% improvement), steroid-sparing effect; improvement in mood and reduction in steroid dependency
Krebs et al.	2010	Clinical Trial (6 weeks)	Wormwood supplementation in UC	Reduction in disease activity and reduction in TNF-α levels	Moderate decrease in blood pressure ($P < 0.002$) with stable renal function
Boswellia serrata					
Gupta et al.	2001	Randomized controlled trial (RCT)	UC patients (Boswellia vs. sulfasalazine)	Efficacy in maintaining UC remission	*Boswellia serrata* extract showed comparable efficacy to sulfasalazine in maintaining remission, with significant symptom improvements in patients

DOI: http://dx.doi.org/10.5772/intechopen.1007705

Author	Year	Type of study	Study design	Primary outcome	Results
Labesque et al.	2008	Animal models	Comparison of LTE_4 excretion in IBD patients vs. controls	Inhibition of 5-lipoxygenase, anti-inflammatory effects	LTE_4 urinary excretion was significantly higher in UC patients than in controls ($P < 0.01$), and boswellic acid selectively inhibited 5-lipoxygenase, showing anti-inflammatory and anti-proliferative properties
Siemoneit et al.	2011	In vitro models	Anti-inflammatory effects of boswellic acids	Identification of mPGES1 as a boswellic acid-interacting protein	β-Boswellic acid (1 mg/kg i.p.) reduced mouse paw edema and PGE_2 levels and the β-BA inhibited lipopolysaccharide-induced PGE_2 biosynthesis without affecting other COX-derived metabolites
Aloe vera					
Langmead et al.	2004	Randomized double-blind study	44 patients with active UC (2:1 *A. vera*)	Clinical response and remission rates	*Aloe vera* gel significantly improved remission (30%), improvement (37%), and clinical response (47%) compared to placebo ($P < 0.05$)
Bahrami et al.	2020	Animal study (acetic acid-induced UC in rats)	Rats pretreated with 50 mg/kg *Aloe vera*	Reduction in inflammation, ulceration, and tissue damage	*Aloe vera* reduced inflammation, ulcers, and tissue damage in UC-induced rats, demonstrating anti-inflammatory effects on the gut mucosa
Germinated barley					
Kanauchi et al.	2003	Clinical trial	Long-term efficacy of GB	Symptom alleviation in UC patients	Significant decrease in clinical activity index ($p < 0.05$), reduction in visible blood in stools, and promote mucosal healing
Hanai et al.	2004	Randomized controlled study	UC patients (intervention and control)	Corticosteroid usage, clinical symptom severity, UC recurrence	Significant decrease in corticosteroid usage after 3 months. After 12 months, patients in the intervention group had lower symptom severity and recurrence rates
Wheatgrass juice (*Triticum aestivum*)					
Arye et al.	2002	Pilot Clinical Study	Effects of wheatgrass juice on UC	Decrease in abdominal pain	Wheatgrass juice reduced rectal bleeding in patients with active UC. Improvement in overall disease severity was observed

Author	Year	Type of study	Study design	Primary outcome	Results
Chamomile					
Menghini et al.	2016	Animal model	Chamomile vs. sulfasalazine comparison	Reduction in myeloperoxidase (MPO) levels	Significant reduction in MPO production observed, significant decrease in IL-6, TNF-α, and NF-kB levels, and as effective as sulfasalazine in reducing inflammation

Table 6.
Summary of evidence on the effects of other botanical remedies in UC patients.

3. Conclusions

Complementary therapies offer promising adjunctive treatments for ulcerative colitis (UC), addressing the limitations of conventional therapies. Probiotics and prebiotics induce remission in mild-to-moderate UC and maintain remission. The anti-inflammatory and immunomodulatory properties of curcumin have demonstrated the potential to induce and maintain remission, especially in patients unresponsive to conventional treatments. Fish oil, rich in omega-3 fatty acids, is effective in protecting the intestinal mucosa. Chinese herbal medicines, such as *Andrographis paniculata* and Indigo Naturalis, along with other botanical remedies like *Artemisia absinthium*, *Boswellia serrata*, *Aloe vera*, germinated barley foodstuff, wheatgrass juice, and chamomile, have shown varying degrees of efficacy in clinical studies. The clinical evidence for these complementary therapies highlights their potential in managing UC, particularly for patients seeking alternatives to conventional treatments.

To fully harness the potential of complementary therapies for ulcerative colitis (UC), future research must prioritize large-scale randomized controlled trials to establish efficacy and safety conclusively. Detailed mechanistic studies are needed to uncover the biological pathways through which these therapies exert their effects. Developing standardized treatment protocols, including precise dosages and administration guidelines, will facilitate their integration into conventional clinical practice. Personalized medicine approaches should be explored to tailor treatments based on individual patient profiles, optimizing therapeutic outcomes. Additionally, fostering interdisciplinary collaboration and increasing funding for research in this area will accelerate the translation of promising findings into clinical applications, ultimately enhancing patient care and expanding the therapeutic arsenal for UC.

Acknowledgements

The author acknowledges the use of ChatGPT for language polishing of the manuscript.

Conflict of interest

The authors declare no conflict of interest.

Declarations

Consent for publication: none.

Acronyms and abbreviations

UC	ulcerative colitis
IBD	inflammatory bowel disease
ASAs	aminosalicylic acids
CAM	complementary and alternative medicine
NF-κB	nuclear factor kappa B
TGF-β	transforming growth factor beta
FOS	fructooligosaccharides
GOS	galactooligosaccharides
XOS	xylooligosaccharides
IL-6	interleukin-6
IL-8	interleukin-8
iNOS	inducible nitric oxide synthase
COX-2	cyclo oxygenase-2
IFN-γ	interferon-γ
MPO	myeloperoxidase
RCT	randomized controlled trial
VSL#3	probiotic mixture
PGE2	prostaglandin-E2

Author details

Vijay Kondreddy[1*], Bhavani Gadiraju[1] and Jhansi Magisetty[2*]

1 Department of Biochemistry, Central University of Punjab, Bathinda, India

2 Department of Zoology, Central University of Punjab, Bathinda, India

*Address all correspondence to: peddireddyvijay@gmail.com
and jhansi.lakshmi@cup.edu.in

References

[1] Jairath V, Feagan BG. Global burden of inflammatory bowel disease. The Lancet Gastroenterology & Hepatology. 2020;**5**:2-3. DOI: 10.1016/S2468-1253(19)30358-9

[2] Danese S, Fiocchi C. Ulcerative colitis. New England Journal of Medicine. 2011;**365**:1713-1725. DOI: 10.1056/NEJMra1102942

[3] Lavelle A, Sokol H. Gut microbiota-derived metabolites as key actors in inflammatory bowel disease. Nature Reviews Gastroenterology & Hepatology. 2020;**17**:223-237. DOI: 10.1038/s41575-019-0258-z

[4] Turner JR. Intestinal mucosal barrier function in health and disease. Nature Reviews Immunology. 2009;**9**:799-809. DOI: 10.1038/nri2653

[5] Zheng T, Wang X, Chen Z, He A, Zheng Z, Liu G. Efficacy of adjuvant curcumin therapy in ulcerative colitis: A meta-analysis of randomized controlled trials. Journal of Gastroenterology and Hepatology. 2020;**35**:722-729. DOI: 10.1111/jgh.14911

[6] Ungaro R, Mehandru S, Allen PB, Peyrin-Biroulet L, Colombel J-F. Ulcerative colitis. The Lancet. 2017;**389**:1756-1770. DOI: 10.1016/S0140-6736(16)32126-2

[7] Carbonnel F, Colombel JF, Filippi J, Katsanos KH, Peyrin-Biroulet L, Allez M, et al. Methotrexate is not superior to placebo for inducing steroid-free remission, but induces steroid-free clinical remission in a larger proportion of patients with ulcerative colitis. Gastroenterology. 2016;**150**:380-388.e384. DOI: 10.1053/j.gastro.2015.10.050

[8] Alatab S, Sepanlou SG, Ikuta K, Vahedi H, Bisignano C, Safiri S, et al. The global, regional, and national burden of inflammatory bowel disease in 195 countries and territories, 1990-2017: A systematic analysis for the Global Burden of Disease Study 2017. The Lancet Gastroenterology & Hepatology. 2020;**5**:17-30. DOI: 10.1016/S2468-1253(19)30333-4

[9] Singh S, Boland BS, Jess T, Moore AA. Management of inflammatory bowel diseases in older adults. The Lancet Gastroenterology & Hepatology. 2023;**8**:368-382. DOI: 10.1016/s2468-1253(22)00358-2

[10] Yanai H, Salomon N, Lahat A. Complementary therapies in inflammatory bowel diseases. Current Gastroenterology Reports. 2016;**18**:62. DOI: 10.1007/s11894-016-0537-6

[11] Lichtenstein GR, Abreu MT, Cohen R, Tremaine W. American Gastroenterological Association Institute technical review on corticosteroids, immunomodulators, and infliximab in inflammatory bowel disease. Gastroenterology. 2006;**130**:940-987. DOI: 10.1053/j.gastro.2006.01.048

[12] Baumgart DC, Sandborn WJ. Inflammatory bowel disease: Clinical aspects and established and evolving therapies. Lancet. 2007;**369**:1641-1657. DOI: 10.1016/s0140-6736(07)60751-x

[13] Le Berre C, Honap S, Peyrin-Biroulet L. Ulcerative colitis. The Lancet. 2023;**402**:571-584. DOI: 10.1016/S0140-6736(23)00966-2

[14] Gomollón F, Dignass A, Annese V, Tilg H, Van Assche G, Lindsay JO, et al. 3rd European evidence-based consensus

on the diagnosis and management of Crohn's disease 2016: Part 1: Diagnosis and medical management. Journal of Crohn's and Colitis. 2016;**11**:3-25. DOI: 10.1093/ecco-jcc/jjw168

[15] Parkes G, Ungaro RC, Danese S, Abreu MT, Arenson E, Zhou W, et al. Correlation of mucosal healing endpoints with long-term clinical and patient-reported outcomes in ulcerative colitis. Journal of Gastroenterology. 2023;**58**:990-1002. DOI: 10.1007/s00535-023-02013-7

[16] Riva A, Rasoulimehrabani H, Cruz-Rubio JM, Schnorr SL, von Baeckmann C, Inan D, et al. Identification of inulin-responsive bacteria in the gut microbiota via multi-modal activity-based sorting. Nature Communications. 2023;**14**:8210. DOI: 10.1038/s41467-023-43448-z

[17] Sanders ME, Merenstein DJ, Reid G, Gibson GR, Rastall RA. Probiotics and prebiotics in intestinal health and disease: From biology to the clinic. Nature Reviews. Gastroenterology & Hepatology. 2019;**16**:605-616. DOI: 10.1038/s41575-019-0173-3

[18] Quigley EMM. Prebiotics and probiotics in digestive health. Clinical Gastroenterology and Hepatology. 2019;**17**:333-344. DOI: 10.1016/j.cgh.2018.09.028

[19] Claus SP. Inulin prebiotic: Is it all about bifidobacteria? Gut. 2017;**66**:1883. DOI: 10.1136/gutjnl-2017-313800

[20] Koleva PT, Valcheva RS, Sun X, Gänzle MG, Dieleman LA. Inulin and fructo-oligosaccharides have divergent effects on colitis and commensal microbiota in HLA-B27 transgenic rats. The British Journal of Nutrition. 2012;**108**:1633-1643. DOI: 10.1017/s0007114511007203

[21] Hoentjen F, Welling GW, Harmsen HJ, Zhang X, Snart J, Tannock GW, et al. Reduction of colitis by prebiotics in HLA-B27 transgenic rats is associated with microflora changes and immunomodulation. Inflammatory Bowel Disease. 2005;**11**:977-985. DOI: 10.1097/01.mib.0000183421.02316.d5

[22] Wang C, Bai J, Wang B, Yu L, Tian F, Zhao J, et al. Stachyose modulates gut microbiota and alleviates DSS-induced ulcerative colitis in mice. Food Science and Human Wellness. 2023;**12**:2211-2220. DOI: 10.1016/j.fshw.2023.03.041

[23] Lunken GR, Tsai K, Schick A, Lisko DJ, Cook L, Vallance BA, et al. Prebiotic enriched exclusive enteral nutrition suppresses colitis via gut microbiome modulation and expansion of anti-inflammatory T cells in a mouse model of colitis. Cellular and Molecular Gastroenterology and Hepatology. 2021;**12**:1251-1266. DOI: 10.1016/j.jcmgh.2021.06.011

[24] Vulevic J, Drakoularakou A, Yaqoob P, Tzortzis G, Gibson GR. Modulation of the fecal microflora profile and immune function by a novel trans-galactooligosaccharide mixture (B-GOS) in healthy elderly volunteers. The American Journal of Clinical Nutrition. 2008;**88**:1438-1446. DOI: 10.3945/ajcn.2008.26242

[25] Casellas F, Borruel N, Torrejón A, Varela E, Antolin M, Guarner F, et al. Oral oligofructose-enriched inulin supplementation in acute ulcerative colitis is well tolerated and associated with lowered faecal calprotectin. Alimentary Pharmacology & Therapeutics. 2007;**25**:1061-1067. DOI: 10.1111/j.1365-2036.2007.03288.x

[26] Suzuki A, Mitsuyama K, Koga H, Tomiyasu N, Masuda J, Takaki K, et al.

Bifidogenic growth stimulator for the treatment of active ulcerative colitis: A pilot study. Nutrition. 2006;**22**:76-81. DOI: 10.1016/j.nut.2005.04.013

[27] Li Z, Li Z, Zhu L, Dai N, Sun G, Peng L, et al. Effects of xylo-oligosaccharide on the gut microbiota of patients with ulcerative colitis in clinical remission. Frontiers in Nutrition. 2021;**8**:778542. DOI: 10.3389/fnut.2021.778542

[28] Liu Y, Cheng Y, Zhang H, Zhou M, Yu Y, Lin S, et al. Integrated cascade nanozyme catalyzes in vivo ROS scavenging for anti-inflammatory therapy. Science Advances. 2020;**6**:eabb2695. DOI: 10.1126/sciadv.abb2695

[29] Kruis W, Fric P, Pokrotnieks J, Lukás M, Fixa B, Kascák M, et al. Maintaining remission of ulcerative colitis with the probiotic Escherichia coli Nissle 1917 is as effective as with standard mesalazine. Gut. 2004;**53**:1617-1623. DOI: 10.1136/gut.2003.037747

[30] Cheifetz AS, Gianotti R, Luber R, Gibson PR. Complementary and alternative medicines used by patients with inflammatory bowel diseases. Gastroenterology. 2017;**152**:415-429.e415. DOI: 10.1053/j.gastro.2016.10.004

[31] Guo Q, Jin Y, Chen X, Ye X, Shen X, Lin M, et al. NF-κB in biology and targeted therapy: New insights and translational implications signal transduction and targeted. Therapy. 2024;**9**:53. DOI: 10.1038/s41392-024-01757-9

[32] Spiller R. Probiotics: An ideal anti-inflammatory treatment for IBS? Gastroenterology. 2005;**128**:783-785. DOI: 10.1053/j.gastro.2005.01.018

[33] Morshedi M, Hashemi R, Moazzen S, Sahebkar A, Hosseinifard E-S. Immunomodulatory and anti-inflammatory effects of probiotics in multiple sclerosis: A systematic review. Journal of Neuroinflammation. 2019;**16**:231. DOI: 10.1186/s12974-019-1611-4

[34] Sartor RB. Therapeutic manipulation of the enteric microflora in inflammatory bowel diseases: Antibiotics, probiotics, and prebiotics. Gastroenterology. 2004;**126**:1620-1633. DOI: 10.1053/j.gastro.2004.03.024

[35] Tursi A, Brandimarte G, Papa A, Giglio A, Elisei W, Giorgetti GM, et al. Treatment of relapsing mild-to-moderate ulcerative colitis with the probiotic VSL#3 as adjunctive to a standard pharmaceutical treatment: A double-blind, randomized, placebo-controlled study. American Journal of Gastroenterology. 2010;**105**:2218-2227. DOI: 10.1038/ajg.2010.218

[36] Miele E, Pascarella F, Giannetti E, Quaglietta L, Baldassano RN, Staiano A. Effect of a probiotic preparation (VSL#3) on induction and maintenance of remission in children with ulcerative colitis. The American Journal of Gastroenterology. 2009;**104**:437-443. DOI: 10.1038/ajg.2008.118

[37] Bibiloni R, Fedorak RN, Tannock GW, Madsen KL, Gionchetti P, Campieri M, et al. VSL#3 probiotic-mixture induces remission in patients with active ulcerative colitis. The American Journal of Gastroenterology. 2005;**100**:1539-1546. DOI: 10.1111/j.1572-0241.2005.41794.x

[38] Tegegne BA, Kebede B. Probiotics, their prophylactic and therapeutic applications in human health development: A review of the literature. Heliyon. 2022;**8**:6. DOI: 10.1016/j.heliyon.2022.e09725

[39] Bohlouli J, Namjoo I, Borzoo-Isfahani M, Hojjati Kermani MA, Balouch Zehi Z, Moravejolahkami AR. Effect of probiotics on oxidative stress and inflammatory status in diabetic nephropathy: A systematic review and meta-analysis of clinical trials. Heliyon. 2021;7:1. DOI: 10.1016/j.heliyon.2021.e05925

[40] Chakraborty A, Mahajan S, Jaiswal SK, Sharma VK. Genome sequencing of turmeric provides evolutionary insights into its medicinal properties. Communications Biology. 2021;**4**:1193. DOI: 10.1038/s42003-021-02720-y

[41] Sugimoto K, Hanai H, Tozawa K, Aoshi T, Uchijima M, Nagata T, et al. Curcumin prevents and ameliorates trinitrobenzene sulfonic acid-induced colitis in mice. Gastroenterology. 2002;**123**:1912-1922. DOI: 10.1053/gast.2002.37050

[42] Hanai H, Iida T, Takeuchi K, Watanabe F, Maruyama Y, Andoh A, et al. Curcumin maintenance therapy for ulcerative colitis: Randomized, multicenter, double-blind, placebo-controlled trial. Clinical Gastroenterology and Hepatology. 2006;**4**:1502-1506. DOI: 10.1016/j.cgh.2006.08.008

[43] Moss AC. Curcumin for maintenance therapy in ulcerative colitis. Clinical Gastroenterology and Hepatology. 2007;**5**:642. DOI: 10.1016/j.cgh.2007.03.002

[44] Ukil A, Maity S, Karmakar S, Datta N, Vedasiromoni JR, Das PK. Curcumin, the major component of food flavour turmeric, reduces mucosal injury in trinitrobenzene sulphonic acid-induced colitis. British Journal of Pharmacology. 2003;**139**:209-218. DOI: 10.1038/sj.bjp.0705241

[45] Jagetia GC, Aggarwal BB. "spicing up" of the immune system by curcumin. Journal of Clinical Immunology. 2007;**27**:19-35. DOI: 10.1007/s10875-006-9066-7

[46] Kumar S, Ahuja V, Sankar MJ, Kumar A, Moss AC. Curcumin for maintenance of remission in ulcerative colitis Cochrane database. Systematic Reviews. 2012;**10**:Cd008424. DOI: 10.1002/14651858.CD008424.pub2

[47] Makrides M, Best K, Yelland L, McPhee A, Zhou S, Quinlivan J, et al. A randomized trial of prenatal n−3 fatty acid supplementation and preterm delivery. New England Journal of Medicine. 2019;**381**:1035-1045. DOI: 10.1056/NEJMoa1816832

[48] Reddy KVK, Naidu KA. Oleic acid, hydroxytyrosol and n-3 fatty acids collectively modulate colitis through reduction of oxidative stress and IL-8 synthesis; in vitro and in vivo studies. International Immunopharmacology. 2016;**35**:29-42. DOI: 10.1016/j.intimp.2016.03.019

[49] Kondreddy VKR, Anikisetty M, Naidu KA. Medium-chain triglycerides and monounsaturated fatty acids potentiate the beneficial effects of fish oil on selected cardiovascular risk factors in rats. The Journal of Nutritional Biochemistry. 2016;**28**:91-102. DOI: 10.1016/j.jnutbio.2015.10.005

[50] de Roos B, Mavrommatis Y, Brouwer IA. Long-chain n-3 polyunsaturated fatty acids: New insights into mechanisms relating to inflammation and coronary heart disease. British Journal of Pharmacology. 2009;**158**:413-428. DOI: 10.1111/j.1476-5381.2009.00189.x

[51] Ma C, Vasu R, Zhang H. The role of long-chain fatty acids in

inflammatory bowel disease. Mediators of Inflammation. 2019;**2019**:8495913. DOI: 10.1155/2019/8495913

[52] Magisetty J, Gadiraju B, Kondreddy V. Genomic analysis in the colon tissues of omega-3 fatty acid-treated rats identifies novel gene signatures implicated in ulcerative colitis. International Journal of Biological Macromolecules. 2024;**258**:128867. DOI: 10.1016/j.ijbiomac.2023.128867

[53] Reddy KVK, Naidu KA. Maternal and neonatal dietary intake of balanced n-6/n-3 fatty acids modulates experimental colitis in young adult rats. European Journal of Nutrition. 2016;**55**:1875-1890. DOI: 10.1007/s00394-015-1004-0

[54] MacLean CH, Mojica WA, Newberry SJ, Pencharz J, Garland RH, Tu W, et al. Systematic review of the effects of n-3 fatty acids in inflammatory bowel disease. The American Journal of Clinical Nutrition. 2005;**82**:611-619. DOI: 10.1093/ajcn.82.3.611

[55] Seidner DL, Lashner BA, Brzezinski A, Banks PLC, Goldblum J, Fiocchi C, et al. An oral supplement enriched with fish oil, soluble fiber, and antioxidants for corticosteroid sparing in ulcerative colitis: A randomized, controlled trial. Clinical Gastroenterology and Hepatology. 2005;**3**:358-369. DOI: 10.1016/S1542-3565(04)00672-X

[56] Masaenah E, Elya B, Setiawan H, Fadhilah Z, Wediasari F, Nugroho GA, et al. Antidiabetic activity and acute toxicity of combined extract of *Andrographis paniculata*, *Syzygium cumini*, and *Caesalpinia sappan*. Heliyon. 2021;**7**:12. DOI: 10.1016/j.heliyon.2021.e08561

[57] Tan Lim AM, Oyong GG, Tan MCS, Chang Shen C, Ragasa CY, Cabrera EC. Quorum quenching activity of *Andrographis paniculata* (Burm f.) Nees andrographolide compounds on metallo-β-lactamase-producing clinical isolates of *Pseudomonas aeruginosa* PA22 and PA247 and their effect on *lasR* gene expression. Heliyon. 2021;**7**:5. DOI: 10.1016/j.heliyon.2021.e07002

[58] Gao Z, Yu C, Liang H, Wang X, Liu Y, Li X, et al. Andrographolide derivative CX-10 ameliorates dextran sulphate sodium-induced ulcerative colitis in mice: Involvement of NF-κB and MAPK signalling pathways. International Immunopharmacology. 2018;**57**:82-90. DOI: 10.1016/j.intimp.2018.02.012

[59] Xia YF, Ye BQ, Li YD, Wang JG, He XJ, Lin X, et al. Andrographolide attenuates inflammation by inhibition of NF-kappa B activation through covalent modification of reduced cysteine 62 of p50. Journal of Immunology. 2004;**173**:4207-4217. DOI: 10.4049/jimmunol.173.6.4207

[60] Sandborn WJ, Targan SR, Byers VS, Rutty DA, Mu H, Zhang X, et al. *Andrographis paniculata* extract (HMPL-004) for active ulcerative colitis. Official Journal of the American College of Gastroenterology |ACG. 2013;**108**:90-98. DOI: 10.1038/ajg.2012.340

[61] Michelsen KS, Wong MH, Ko B, Thomas LS, Dhall D, Targan SR. HMPL-004 (*Andrographis paniculata* extract) prevents development of murine colitis by inhibiting T-cell proliferation and TH1/TH17 responses. Inflammatory Bowel Disease. 2013;**19**:151-164. DOI: 10.1002/ibd.22983

[62] Matsuno Y, Umeno J, Hirano A, Fuyuno Y, Nagasue T, Fujioka S, et al. Maintenance efficacy of oral Indigo Naturalis for ulcerative colitis: A single-center, open-label, randomized, controlled study. Gastroenterology. 2024;**166**:S12. DOI: 10.1053/j.gastro.2023.11.052

[63] Hiraide T, Teratani T, Kataoka M, Endo J, Sano M, Hakamata Y, et al. Abstract 640: Indigo Naturalis, a promising herbal medicine for ulcerative colitis, can induce experimental pulmonary arterial hypertension via aryl hydrocarbon pathway. Circulation Research. 2019;**125**:A640-A640. DOI: 10.1161/res.125.suppl_1.640

[64] Matsuno Y, Hirano A, Okamoto Y, Fuyuno Y, Fujioka S, Umeno J, et al. P048 short- and long-term outcome of patients treated with indigo naturalis for inflammatory bowel disease: A single center retrospective study. Gastroenterology. 2019;**156**:S34-S35. DOI: 10.1053/j.gastro.2019.01.103

[65] Yokote A, Imazu N, Umeno J, Kawasaki K, Fujioka S, Fuyuno Y, et al. Ferroptosis in the colon epithelial cells as a therapeutic target for ulcerative colitis. Journal of Gastroenterology. 2023;**58**:868-882. DOI: 10.1007/s00535-023-02016-4

[66] Kawai S, Iijima H, Shinzaki S, Hiyama S, Yamaguchi T, Araki M, et al. Indigo Naturalis ameliorates murine dextran sodium sulfate-induced colitis via aryl hydrocarbon receptor activation. Journal of Gastroenterology. 2017;**52**:904-919. DOI: 10.1007/s00535-016-1292-z

[67] Li H, Zhao L, Zhang B, Jiang Y, Wang X, Guo Y, et al. A network pharmacology approach to determine active compounds and action mechanisms of Ge-gen-Qin-Lian decoction for treatment of type 2 diabetes. Evidence-based Complementary and Alternative Medicine. 2014;**2014**:495840. DOI: 10.1155/2014/495840

[68] Naganuma M, Sugimoto S, Mitsuyama K, Kobayashi T, Yoshimura N, Ohi H, et al. Efficacy of indigo naturalis in a multicenter randomized controlled trial of patients with ulcerative colitis. Gastroenterology. 2018;**154**:935-947. DOI: 10.1053/j.gastro.2017.11.024

[69] Wang Y, Liu L, Guo Y, Mao T, Shi R, Li J. Effects of indigo naturalis on colonic mucosal injuries and inflammation in rats with dextran sodium sulphate-induced ulcerative colitis. Experimental and Therapeutic Medicine. 2017;**14**:1327-1336. DOI: 10.3892/etm.2017.4701

[70] Algieri F, Rodriguez-Nogales A, Rodriguez-Cabezas ME, Risco S, Ocete MA, Galvez J. Botanical drugs as an emerging strategy in inflammatory bowel disease: A review. Mediators of Inflammation. 2015;**2015**:179616. DOI: 10.1155/2015/179616

[71] Wang KS, Li J, Wang Z, Mi C, Ma J, Piao LX, et al. Artemisinin inhibits inflammatory response via regulating NF-κB and MAPK signaling pathways. Immunopharmacology an Immunotoxicology. 2017;**39**:28-36. DOI: 10.1080/08923973.2016.1267744

[72] Jin Q, Liu T, Chen D, Yang L, Mao H, Ma F, et al. Therapeutic potential of artemisinin and its derivatives in managing kidney diseases. Frontiers in Pharmacology. 2023;**14**:1097206. DOI: 10.3389/fphar.2023.1097206

[73] Krebs S, Omer TN, Omer B. Wormwood (*Artemisia absinthium*) suppresses tumour necrosis factor alpha and accelerates healing in patients with Crohn's disease – A controlled clinical trial. Phytomedicine. 2010;**17**:305-309. DOI: 10.1016/j.phymed.2009.10.013

[74] Omer B, Krebs S, Omer H, Noor TO. Steroid-sparing effect of wormwood (*Artemisia absinthium*) in Crohn's disease: A double-blind placebo-controlled study. Phytomedicine. 2007;**14**:87-95. DOI: 10.1016/j.phymed.2007.01.001

[75] Krebs S, Omer B, Omer TN, Fliser D. Wormwood (*Artemisia absinthium*) for poorly responsive early-stage IgA nephropathy: A pilot uncontrolled trial. American Journal of Kidney Diseases. 2010;**56**:1095-1099. DOI: 10.1053/j.ajkd.2010.06.025

[76] Alharbi SA, Asad M, Abdelsalam KEA, Chandy S, Ibrahim MA. Frankincense extract protects against testicular damage through augmentation of antioxidant defense mechanisms and modulation of apoptotic genes expression. Scientific Reports. 2022;**12**:12625. DOI: 10.1038/s41598-022-16920-x

[77] Wang H, Syrovets T, Kess D, Büchele B, Hainzl H, Lunov O, et al. Targeting NF-κB with a natural Triterpenoid alleviates skin inflammation in a mouse model of Psoriasis1. The Journal of Immunology. 2009;**183**:4755-4763. DOI: 10.4049/jimmunol.0900521

[78] Stanke-Labesque F, Pofelski J, Moreau-Gaudry A, Bessard G, Bonaz B. Urinary leukotriene E4 excretion: A biomarker of inflammatory bowel disease activity. Inflammatory Bowel Diseases. 2008;**14**:769-774. DOI: 10.1002/ibd.20403

[79] Siemoneit U, Koeberle A, Rossi A, Dehm F, Verhoff M, Reckel S, et al. Inhibition of microsomal prostaglandin E2 synthase-1 as a molecular basis for the anti-inflammatory actions of boswellic acids from frankincense. British Journal of Pharmacology. 2011;**162**:147-162. DOI: 10.1111/j.1476-5381.2010.01020.x

[80] Gupta I, Parihar A, Malhotra P, Gupta S, Lüdtke R, Safayhi H, et al. Effects of gum resin of Boswellia serrata in patients with chronic colitis. Planta Medica. 2001;**67**:391-395. DOI: 10.1055/s-2001-15802

[81] Langhorst J, Wulfert H, Lauche R, Klose P, Cramer H, Dobos GJ, et al. Systematic review of complementary and alternative medicine treatments in inflammatory bowel diseases. Journal of Crohn's and Colitis. 2014;**9**:86-106. DOI: 10.1093/ecco-jcc/jju007

[82] Langmead L, Feakins RM, Goldthorpe S, Holt H, Tsironi E, De Silva A, et al. Randomized, double-blind, placebo-controlled trial of oral aloe vera gel for active ulcerative colitis. Alimentary Pharmacology & Therapeutics. 2004;**19**:739-747. DOI: 10.1111/j.1365-2036.2004.01902.x

[83] Bahrami G, Malekshahi H, Miraghaee S, Madani H, Babaei A, Mohammadi B, et al. Protective and therapeutic effects of aloe Vera gel on ulcerative colitis induced by acetic acid in rats. Clinical Nutrition Research. 2020;**9**:223-234. DOI: 10.7762/cnr.2020.9.3.223

[84] Kanauchi O, Suga T, Tochihara M, Hibi T, Naganuma M, Homma T, et al. Treatment of ulcerative colitis by feeding with germinated barley foodstuff: First report of a multicenter open control trial. Journal of Gastroenterology. 2002;**37**(Suppl. 14):67-72. DOI: 10.1007/bf03326417

[85] Kanauchi O, Mitsuyama K, Andoh A. Chapter 39 - germinated barley foodstuff dampens inflammatory bowel disease. In: Watson RR, Preedy VR, Zibadi S, editors. Wheat and Rice in Disease Prevention and Health. San Diego: Academic Press; 2014. pp. 507-519

[86] Kanauchi O, Mitsuyama K, Homma T, Takahama K, Fujiyama Y, Andoh A, et al. Treatment of ulcerative colitis patients by long-term administration of germinated barley foodstuff: Multi-center open trial. International Journal of Molecular Medicine. 2003;**12**:701-704

[87] Hanai H, Kanauchi O, Mitsuyama K, Andoh A, Takeuchi K, Takayuki I, et al. Germinated barley foodstuff prolongs remission in patients with ulcerative colitis. International Journal of Molecular Medicine. 2004;**13**:643-647

[88] Ben-Arye E, Goldin E, Wengrower D, Stamper A, Kohn R, Berry E. Wheat grass juice in the treatment of active distal ulcerative colitis: A randomized double-blind placebo-controlled trial. Scandinavian Journal of Gastroenterology. 2002;**37**:444-449. DOI: 10.1080/003655202317316088

[89] Al-Dabbagh B, Elhaty IA, Elhaw M, Murali C, Al Mansoori A, Awad B, et al. Antioxidant and anticancer activities of chamomile (*Matricaria recutita* L.). BMC Research Notes. 2019;**12**:3. DOI: 10.1186/s13104-018-3960-y

[90] Langhorst J, Koch AK, Voiss P, Dobos GJ, Rueffer A. Distinct patterns of short-chain fatty acids during flare in patients with ulcerative colitis under treatment with mesalamine or a herbal combination of myrrh, chamomile flowers, and coffee charcoal: Secondary analysis of a randomized controlled trial. European Journal of Gastroenterology & Hepatology. 2020;**32**:175-180. DOI: 10.1097/meg.0000000000001582

[91] Menghini L, Ferrante C, Leporini L, Recinella L, Chiavaroli A, Leone S, et al. An Hydroalcoholic chamomile extract modulates inflammatory and immune response in HT29 cells and isolated rat Colon. Phytotherapy Research. 2016;**30**:1513-1518. DOI: 10.1002/ptr.5655